AIDS
MUSCULOSKELETAL MANIFESTATIONS

AIDS
MUSCULOSKELETAL MANIFESTATIONS

Jamshid Tehranzadeh, M.D.
and
Lynne S. Steinbach, M.D.

WARREN H. GREEN, INC.
St. Louis, Missouri, U.S.A.

Published by

WARREN H. GREEN, INC.
8356 Olive Boulevard
St. Louis, Missouri 63132 U.S.A.

ISBN No. 0-87527-5095

Printed in the United States of America

FOREWORD

Infection produced by human immunodeficiency virus (HIV) and the resulting autoimmune deficiency syndrome (AIDS) represent the most important of medical problems, affecting ever increasing numbers of adults and children. No organ system escapes the potentially devastating effects of AIDS, and its influence on the musculoskeletal system can be profound. Despite this, no single reference has existed to which an interested physician could refer to learn more about the musculoskeletal abnormalities of AIDS. To correct this deficiency, two leading bone radiologists, Jamshid Tehranzadeh and Lynne S. Steinbach, with the help of six other physicians, have combined their efforts to provide a work that is both timely and important. The two editors and their contributors have examined every facet of musculoskeletal involvement in AIDS, including soft tissue, articular, and osseous infection and inflammation, neoplasms, and bone marrow alterations, and they have done so in a well-organized and easy to read book. Such involvement is illustrated in exquisite fashion using routine and advanced imaging methods, including computed tomography and magnetic resonance. Selected references are included to guide the reader who might wish to seek further information on the subject.

Although many physicians are aware that AIDS can lead to a variety of musculoskeletal problems, most, including this radiologist, are not familiar with the many ways that this syndrome can be displayed. The information contained in this work provides practical clues that aid in the correct diagnosis of these many musculoskeletal manifestations and, equally important, gives insight into pathogenesis and appropriate imaging assessment. As such, it represents a most important contribution to the medical literature and essential reading to those professionals involved in the diagnosis and treatment of this syndrome.

The authors are to be commended for addressing a subject that largely had been ignored and providing a precise source of information. It is a first-rate accomplishment and one for which I am honored to be able to write this foreword.

Donald L. Resnick, M.D.

DEDICATION

This book is dedicated to all children and adults who are victims of this disease, with the hope of an eminent cure.

Jamshid Tehranzadeh
Lynne S. Steinbach

PREFACE

Human immunodeficiency virus (HIV) infection has reached epidemic proportions. It is no longer merely a disease of male homosexuals or hemophiliacs. According to the latest report from the Center for Disease Control on March 31, 1993, the cumulative number of AIDS cases reported to CDC is 289,328. Among these, 252,363 are men and 32,477 cases are women. Through the same time period, 4,488 cases were reported in children under the age of thirteen years.

Autoimmune Deficiency Syndrome (AIDS) is a multisystem disease that decreases the body's defense mechanism and predisposes infected individuals to a variety of opportunistic infections, immune-related neoplasms, anemia, myositis, and arthritis. As a multiorgan disease, the pulmonary and central nervous systems are primarily involved; however, gastrointestinal, genitourinary, cutaneous, musculoskeletal, and other systems are affected.

Although rheumatic complaints and problems have been reported up to 65-72% in AIDS patients, little has been written about the skeletal and soft tissue manifestations of HIV infection. The knowledge about the musculoskeletal manifestations of this disease is important both to clinicians and to radiologists. The information is also beneficial for HIV-positive patients and millions of health care workers taking care of this patient population.

This book critically reviews our materials and current knowledge of musculoskeletal manifestations of this disease and will keep the reader up to date on this subject. "Musculoskeletal Manifestations of Acquired Immune Deficiency Syndrome" systemically reviews in separate chapters each of the musculoskeletal abnormalities associated with AIDS, including infection, tuberculosis, bacillary angiomatosis, lymphoma, Kaposi sarcoma, arthritis, myositis, and other miscellaneous conditions using extensive current literature citations and superb illustrative case presentations. An attempt was made to use state-of-the-art modalities in imaging, such as computed tomography and magnetic resonance imaging, as well as conventional radiography and scintigraphy to depict various osseous, articular, and soft tissue changes in these patients. The case material is the product of over twelve years of observations of the authors of the book, from five major university hospitals located in large metropolitan areas in the United States, as well as referrals from other locations.

The first step in solving any problem is to diagnose and recognize the problem. It is highly imperative for physicians in general and radiologists, in particular, to know and look for the different clinical and imaging manifestations of AIDS.

Jamshid Tehranzadeh

EDITORS:

JAMSHID TEHRANZADEH, M.D.
Professor of Radiology and Orthopaedics
Director of Musculoskeletal Radiology
Department of Radiological Sciences
University of California Irvine
Irvine, California

LYNNE S. STEINBACH, M.D.
Associate Professor of Clinical Radiology
Department of Radiology
University of California San Francisco
San Francisco, California

CONTRIBUTORS:

DEBRA BUTLER, M.D.
Resident of Radiology, Department of Radiological Sciences
University of California Irvine
Irvine, California

CHRIS CASSADY, M.D.
Chief Resident of Radiology, Department of Radiological Sciences
University of California Irvine
Irvine, California

JAMES L. FLECKENSTEIN, M.D.
Director, Neuro MR, Department of Radiology
University of Texas Southwestern Medical Center
Dallas, Texas

MAMED MESGARZADEH, M.D.
Professor of Radiology, Department of Diagnostic Imaging
Temple University
Philadelphia, Pennsylvania

LYNNE S. STEINBACH, M.D.
Associate Professor of Clinical Radiology, Department of Radiology
University of California San Francisco
San Francisco, California

JAMSHID TEHRANZADEH, M.D.
Professor of Radiology and Orthopaedics,
Director of Musculoskeletal Radiology
University of California Irvine
Irvine, California

MICHAEL WENGER, M.D.
Chief Resident of Radiology, Department of Radiology
University of California Irvine
Irvine, California

CAROL WONG, M.D.
Resident of Radiology, Department of Radiology
University of California Irvine
Irvine, California

TABLE OF CONTENTS

ACKNOWLEDGEMENTS

I would like to acknowledge the memory of the late Mr. Warren Green, who originally asked me to write this book, and the efforts of Ms. Joyce Green, who made it happen. I would also like to thank my coeditor, Lynne S. Steinbach, and all of the contributors, Debra Butler, Chris Cassady, James Fleckenstein, Mamed Mesgarzadeh, Michael Wenger, and Carol Wong. My personal thanks go to Akbar Bonakdarpour, Anne Brower, Murray Dalinka, Jack Edeiken, Deborah Forrester, Richard Friedenberg, Gary Ghahremani, Harry Genant, Richard Gold, Theodore Keats, Henry Lerner, Joseph Mirra, Alex Norman, Eric Radin, Donald Resnick, and Lee Rogers for their support and encouragement. My special thanks to Betty Trent for preparation of the manuscripts of this book and to James Ranson for his photographic assistance.

Jamshid Tehranzadeh

AIDS
MUSCULOSKELETAL MANIFESTATIONS

CHAPTER 1:

MUSCULOSKELETAL INFECTION IN HIV-POSITIVE PATIENTS

Jamshid Tehranzadeh, M.D.
Mamed Mesgarzadeh, M.D.

INTRODUCTION

According to the latest report from the Center for Disease Control in March 1993, the cumulative number of acquired immune deficiency syndrome (AIDS) cases reported was 289,320. Of these, 182,275 persons died from this disease. The highest number of patients (132,197) are diagnosed between the ages of 30 to 39. According to the same source, Caucasians have the highest number of AIDS cases in this country, followed by Blacks and Hispanics. New York reported the highest number of AIDS patients, followed by California and Florida. The majority of AIDS cases are seen among male homosexuals (160,345), IV drug abusers (65,778), male homosexuals who are also drug abusers (18,041), and hemophiliacs (2,519) (1). Worldwide, perhaps 5 million persons have been infected with HIV-1, or the related retrovirus, HIV-2 (3). An additional 1 to 1.5 million Americans have been infected with the human immunodeficiency virus (HIV) (2). Most HIV-infected persons will develop AIDS (4,5).

The first cases of AIDS were reported by Gottlieb in 1981 (6). A concentrated effort was made to identify the etiologic agent of AIDS and to describe the various opportunistic infections and the neoplasms associated with this syndrome. Reports of patients who had no known cause for a cellular immunodeficiency and who developed Pneumocystis Carinii pneumonia, candidiasis and/or Kaposi's sarcoma dominated the early literature on AIDS. Homosexual or bisexual men, intravenous drug abusers, hemophiliacs, recipients of blood transfusions, and Haitians were originally identified as high-risk groups as well as heterosexuals having sexual contact with persons at high risk. In 1984, a new human retrovirus with a tropism for T-cell lymphocyte was found to be the causative agent of AIDS and the AIDS-related complex (ARC) (7-10). It was termed the human immuno T-cell lymphotrophic virus type III/lymphadenopathy-associated virus (HTLV III/LAV) or, more recently, the human immunodeficiency virus (HIV) (7-11). Indeed, it is the ability of HIV both to grow in and to destroy T-helper lymphocytes that render the immune system unable to perform its task of host defense (12). Therefore, the hallmark of AIDS is a disturbance in T-cell mediated immunity. These T-cells carry on their surface a glycoprotein molecule called CD4, which has been shown to bind the envelope glycoprotein of HIV. The destruction of CD4-bearing lymphocytes probably accounts for the immunosuppressive effect of the virus. The frequency of complications is directly related to the severity of the immunosuppression and is highest in the patient with a CD4+ (helper) lymphocyte count less than 200/μL (13). It has recently been recognized that the CD4 molecule is also present at lower density, on cells other than helper T-cells. Some monocytes and macrophages as well as B lymphocytes carry CD4 (12).

The clinical spectrum of HIV disease ranges from the asymptomatic state to full-blown AIDS. The term AIDS-related complex (ARC), which is no longer used, refers to patients who present with generalized lymphadenopathy or constitutional symptoms; these patients fall between the two extremes of the spectrum (12). AIDS affects multiple organs, including the pulmonary, gastrointestinal, renal, neurologic, dermatologic, cardiac, ocular, and musculoskeletal systems (12).

Pulmonary Infections

Immune dysfunction in AIDS patients is directly related to CD4+ cell count, the main target of the human immunodeficiency virus (14,15). Preferential involvement of CD4 cells largely accounts for the types of infections seen in AIDS patients as well as the likely sequence and probability with which these complications will arise. For example, Pneumocystis carinii pneumonia, which is the commonest pulmonary infection in AIDS patients (60-80% of the cases), is often found in patients with a CD4+ cell count greater than 100 cells/mm^3, whereas infection with Mycobacterium avium complex and cytomegalovirus typically occurs only in patients whose CD4+ cell count falls below 50 cells/mm^3 (15).

Different radiologic pulmonary manifestations are seen in AIDS patients. An infected lung in an AIDS patient with a normal chest radiographic pattern is mostly caused by P. carinii pneumonia. This organism is also the responsible agent for most diffuse infiltrative radiographic patterns seen in AIDS patients. Pyogenic bacteria is the commonest cause of focal infiltrates in HIV-positive patients. Although a nodular pattern in the lung of an HIV-positive patient has many causes, such as septic emboli, Mycobacterium tuberculosis (M. tuberculosis), fungal infection and lymphoma, Kaposi sarcoma (KS) should be highly considered. Hilar adenopathy is often due to M. tuberculosis, fungal infection or

KS. Association of pleural effusion in HIV-positive patients may be seen with KS, M. tuberculosis, fungal, pyogenic infection, and non-Hodgkin's lymphoma, and is uncommon with P. carinii pneumonia (15).

Gastrointestinal Infections

Many patients with HIV disease who have not yet progressed to AIDS are chronically ill with a wasting-like syndrome that often includes diarrhea (16,17). In the absence of evidence of an opportunistic infection or opportunistic tumor to explain their gastrointestinal symptomatology, the diagnosis of HIV enteropathy is established. Imaging abnormalities of the gastrointestinal tract are indicative of a diagnosis other than HIV enteropathy, and opportunistic infections should be suspected (17). Candida albicans is the opportunistic organism that most commonly involves the gastrointestinal tract in patients with AIDS. Candida esophagitis in an HIV-positive patient constitutes a diagnosis of clinical AIDS (17-20). Other causes of esophagitis in AIDS patients are herpes simplex and cytomegalovirus (CMV) (19). CMV colitis occurs frequently in AIDS patients (17,21). M. tuberculosis can also cause disease in the gastrointestinal tract in AIDS patients (17).

Although a clear tendency exists among AIDS patients for developing opportunistic fungal, protozoan, mycobacterial or viral infections rather than pyogenic agents, systemic bacterial infections such as disseminated streptococcal infection may occur, which can be unusually severe and affect multiple visceral organs (22).

Infection of Nervous System

Neurological manifestation is seen in 10% of AIDS patients, and 50-60% of patients infected with HIV experience neurologic dysfunction during the course of the illness (3,23,24). HIV-1 infection can directly or indirectly cause AIDS-dementia complex, HIV-encephalitis/leukoencephalopathy, vascular myelopathy, neuropathy, myopathy.

Opportunistic microorganisms affecting the CNS of AIDS patients include toxoplasmosis, mycobacteria, spirochetes, aspergillus, candida, cryptococcus, and treponema pallidum. Others include viral, cytomegalovirus (CMV), herpes simplex, herpes zoster, and progressive multifocal leukoencephalopathy (PML). Neoplasms include lymphoma and Kaposi sarcoma. Vascular lesions consist of non-inflammatory vasculopathy and granulomatous angiitis. The neurologic changes in children include basal ganglion calcification, neuroatrophy, corticospinal tract degeneration, and microcephaly (3).

Musculoskeletal Infections

Musculoskeletal infections in HIV-positive patients are relatively uncommon compared to other organ systems. However, AIDS patients are prone to both common and opportunistic agents (25), often because of the host's inability to respond. Clinical presentation may be delayed and response to therapy is commonly suboptimal, producing chronic or borderline subclinical diseases (25).

It is of interest that opportunistic infections were not seen at all in a study of 560 HIV-positive patients by Spencer, et al (26,27). Staph aureus, which is the most common cause of musculoskeletal infection in non-immunocompromised patients (28), remains the leading cause of bone and soft tissue infection in HIV-positive patients. A variety of soft tissue and osteoarticular infections have been reported in AIDS patients. These can be divided as follows:

Musculoskeletal Infections

- A. Soft tissue infection
  1. Cellulitis and lymphedema
  2. Myonecrosis, pyomyositis and soft tissue abscess
- B. Osteoarticular Infection
  1. Osteomyelitis
  2. Discitis and spondylitis
  3. Septic arthritis
  4. Septic bursitis

A. Soft Tissue Infection

A full spectrum of soft tissue infection and inflammation can be seen in HIV-positive patients.

1. Cellulitis and Lymphedema. Cellulitis represents inflammation of the skin and subcutaneous tissue. Cellulitis is usually clinically detectable, especially in the AIDS patient, but superficial primary cellulitis and cellulitis associated with deep infection are difficult to distinguish (25). Owing to its inherent limitations, conventional radiography cannot show soft tissue and fascial layers and generally does not show early osseous changes (25). Cellulitis creates inflammation and consequently edema of the subcutaneous fat without creating a soft tissue mass (Fig. 1). On CT examination the density of subcutaneous fat rises from 90 to 120 H.U. to attenuation numbers closer to that of soft tissue (25). Normally, on MRI fat is bright on TIWI (T1-weighted image) and becomes slightly darker on the T2WI (T2-weighted image). Inflammation and edema causes a decrease in the signal intensity of fat on T1WI and increased signal intensity on T2WI (28). Cellulitis may lead to inflammation in muscle causing myositis, pyomyositis, fasciitis, vascular thrombosis (Fig. 1), and lymphedema.

Lymphedema can also be primary or associated with more proximal obstruction or destruction. The engorged tissues and stagnant lymphatic fluid provide excellent culture media for streptococcal or other secondary infections. A subcutaneous reticulated or honeycomb pattern can be seen on CT examination. The fibrous septa have the low attenuation of soft tissues (20-30 H.U.) and are superimposed against a background of residual fatty subcutaneous densities and normal deep muscle layers (25).

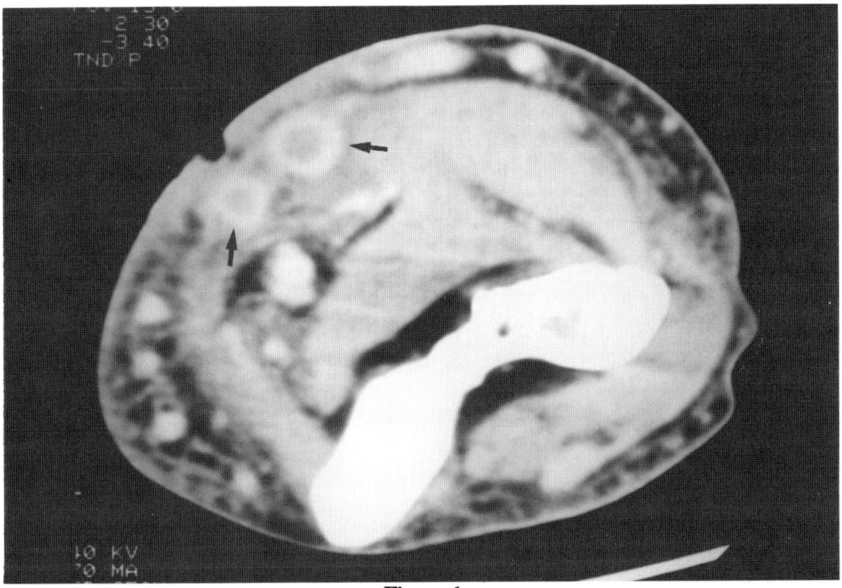

Figure 1

Soft tissue infection. 40-year-old HIV-positive male with antecubital ulcer. CT scan with IV contrast (soft tissue window) shows soft tissue ulcer and edema with brachial artery and vein thrombosis (arrows). Note subcutaneous pus collection, inflammation and edema.

MRI, CT or scintigraphy play an important role in the diagnosis and extent of soft tissue infection changes, myositis, myonecrosis, pyomyositis, fascitis, and soft tissue abscess (Figs. 2 & 3). Sequelae such as periostitis and osteomyelitis can also be successfully imaged and evaluated with these modalities (28). Other diagnostic considerations in HIV-infected patients with focal calf pain and swelling include HIV related "hyperalgesic pseudothrombophlebitis" (29,30). For more information on muscular changes in AIDS, please refer to Chapter 4.

2. Pyomyositis, Myonecrosis and Soft Tissue Abscess.

Pyomyositis. Pyomyositis is pyogenic infection of muscle, most commonly caused by staph aureus (Fig. 2) (Table 1). It is a common disease in the tropics, however, it is rare in the continental United States. A large number of cases of pyomyositis have been described in association with HIV infection (30-50). Other microorganisms including cryptococcus (41), M. tuberculosis (31,42), and streptococcus pyogenes (31) have been reported (Fig. 3). Group A B-hemolytic streptococci have been reported to cause a more progressive and malignant pyomyositis (40). Defects of neutrophil function may contribute to the development of staphylococcal pyomyositis in some HIV-infected patients (30). Polymorphonuclear leukocytes from HIV-infected patients frequently manifest decreased chemotaxis (51-58).

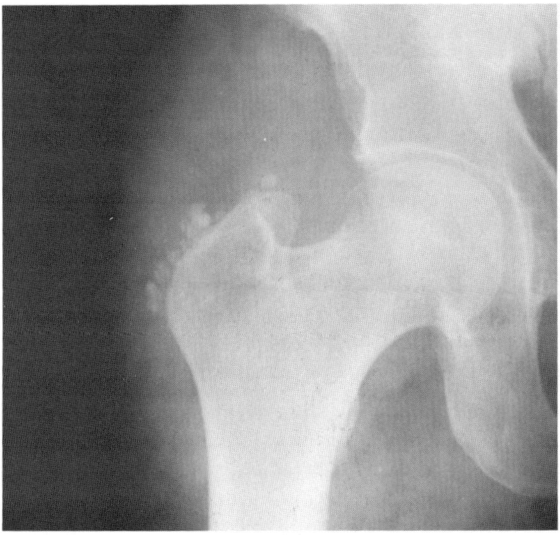

Figure 2-A

Soft tissue abscess. 40 year-old man presenting with a soft tissue abscess of the right gluteal region. Aspiration revealed staph aureus. Plain radiograph of the right hip shows a soft tissue mass with multiple round, small calcific densities in the greater trochanteric region.

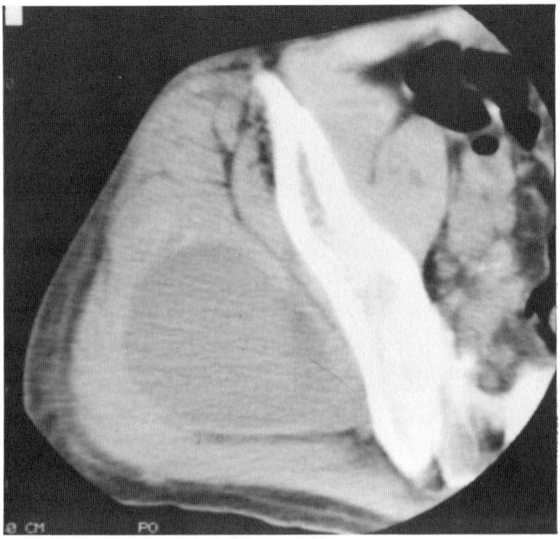

Figure 2-B

CT scan (soft tissue window) of the right hemipelvis shows a well-marginated, oval low-density mass in the gluteal area.

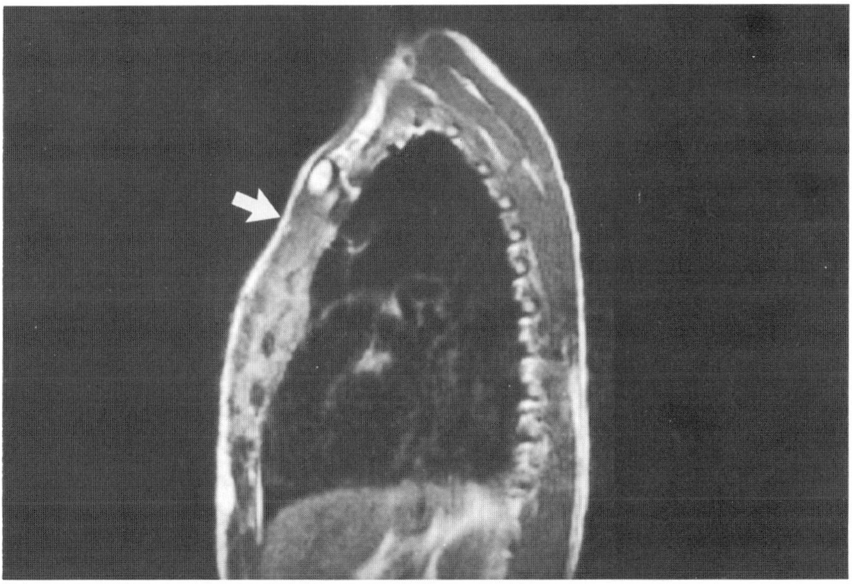

Figure 3-A

Chest wall infection. 30-year old HIV-positive man with chest wall nocardia asteroides abscess. (From Lynne S. Steinbach et al.: Radiology 1993; 186:833-838, with permission.) Parasagittal T1-weighted image (TR 500/TE 30) shows a mass to the left of the sternum in the anterior chest wall (arrow). The mass has low signal intensity on this image.

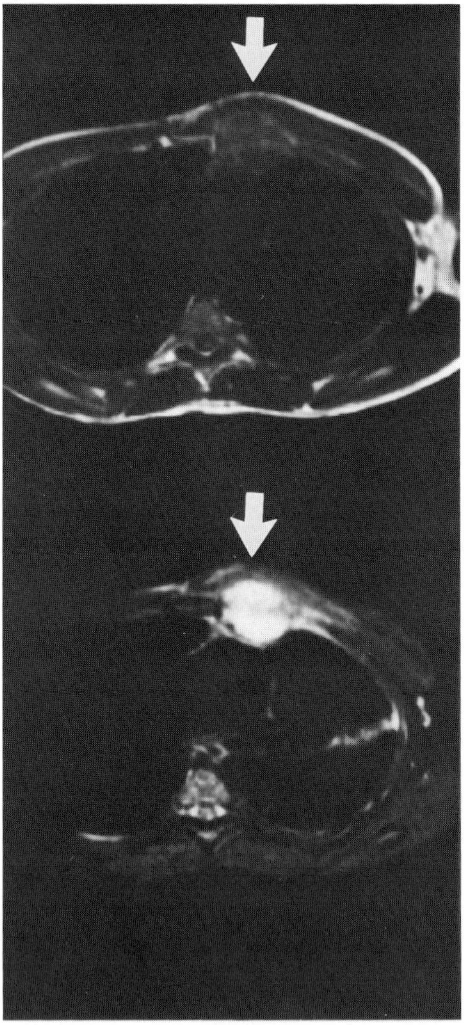

Figure 3-B

30-year old HIV-positive man with chest wall nocardia asteroides abscess. (From Lynne S. Steinbach: Radiology 1993; 186:833-838.) Axial T1-weighted image (TR 500/TE 30) (Top) and STIR (TR 1500/TE 30/TI 95) (bottom) images demonstrate a mass to the left of the sternum in the anterior chest wall (arrow). The mass has low signal intensity on T1-weighted image and high signal intensity on the STIR image.

Different theories have evolved to explain the discordance of geographic incidence and why muscle tissue, which is normally resistant to infection, is affected. Tissue parasites, viruses, spirochetes, and nutritional imbalances have all been described as possible etiologic factors, however, none of these have been shown conclusively to play a role (40). The role of antecedent trauma has been reported to occur in 25-70% of the patients. The possible explanation for tropical pyomyositis may be that people in these areas often walk barefoot and have a high incidence of repetitive minor foot trauma which may serve as foci for a silent pyoderma and a consequent bacteremia (40). Pyomyositis can occur in patients with other immunodeficiencies such as diabetes, Felty's syndrome, and lymphocytic leukemia (40). Myonecrosis initiated by tissue anoxia or trauma, especially when contaminated with foreign material, may lead to pyomyositis and finally muscle abscess. The predominance of non-clostridial myonecrosis in AIDS patients reflects the increasing number of IV drug abusers affected with AIDS. These patients traumatize their muscles and fail to observe sterile technique and occasionally have a prolonged state of stupor and immobility; more than one risk factor may be involved. Myonecrotic muscle is enlarged and has a decreased attenuation value on CT examination compatible with that of edema. A localized intramuscular collection of fluid or gas may be seen. Intramuscular gas may reflect clostridial infection (25). IV contrast material on CT or IV Gadolinium on MRI differentiates between normal (vascularized) muscle and myonecrotic tissue which does not enhance and may help define the abscess (25,31).

An unusual case of Fournier's gangrene of the scrotum in a 33-year-old IV drug abuser with AIDS has been reported (59). Fournier's gangrene is a form of fulminant necrotizing fascitis caused by a synergistic polymicrobial bacterial infection of subcutaneous tissues, which rapidly spreads along the fascial planes.

Clinical manifestations of pyomyositis have three stages (60). The first stage is where pain is localized in one muscle group. There is a woody hardened area of induration with localized pain and low-grade fever. There may be a mild leukocytosis, but needle aspiration will not reveal any pus. In the second stage or so-called "suppurative" stage, pain, fever and edema of the affected muscle is noted in 90% of patients. Needle aspiration at this stage shows a thick, yellow pus. In the third or "late" stage, patients often appear septic and toxic. A fluctuant abscess may be noted and the entire muscle may be replaced by pus. This may be followed by fulminant septicemia and death (40). In the first and second stages of the disease, the diagnosis may be mistaken for a variety of conditions such as cellulitis, muscle tear, hematoma, appendicitis, arthritis, thrombophlebitis, or tumor (40,60). MRI has proven to be very useful in imaging and diagnosis of this disease. For further information regarding imaging of pyomyositis and muscle changes in AIDS, please refer to Chapter 4.

TABLE 1. PYOMYOSITIS IN AIDS PATIENTS (REVIEW OF LITERATURE)

Author	Ref. No.	No. of Cases	Microorganism
Fleckenstein	31	7	5 Staph aureus 1 Strep pyogenes 1 Mycobacteria tuberculosis
Steinbach	27	3	2 Staph aureus 1 Nocardia asteroides
Widrow	32, 33	5	4 Staph aureus C. freundii
Schwartzman	30	5	5 Staph aureus
Thomas	34	2	2 Staph aureus
Blumberg	35	2	2 Staph aureus
Balachandran	36	2	2 Staph aureus
Wolf	37	1	1 Staph aureus
Rodgers	38	1	1 Staph aureus
Wu	39	1	1 Staph aureus septicemia and rhabdomyolysis
Gardiner	40	1	1 Staph aureus (infant)
Wrzoleck	41	2	2 Cryptococcus
Pouchot	42	1	1 Tuberculous polymyositis
Gaut	43	1	1 Staph aureus
Vartian	44	1	1 Staph aureus
Raphael	45	1	1 Staph aureus
Victor	46	1	1 Staph aureus
Elsing	47	1	—
Belec	48	1	—
Watts	49	1	—
Hughes	50	1	1 Salmonella enteritidis

B. Osteoarticular Infection

1. Osteomyelitis. Osteomyelitis, which refers to the infection of bone and its marrow cavity, is relatively uncommon in HIV-positive patients (27,50,61-80) (Figs. 4-8) (Table 2). Staph aureus is the most common cause of osteomyelitis. The hematogenous route may be the most common source of osteomyelitis, especially in IV drug abusers. In Munoz-Fernandez' series (62) of 556 HIV-positive patients, three reported cases of osteomyelitis were all IV drug abusers. In this series the involved sites included wrist, tibia and femoral head. In Spencer's series of 560 HIV-positive patients, 12 cases of osteomyelitis were identified. Staph aureus was the leading cause of osteomyelitis, followed by salmonella (26). In Steinbach's series (27), two cases of staph aureus osteomyelitis, one in the tibia and the second in the rib, were noted. Nocardia asteroides was the cause of soft tissue and bone infection in the thoracic cage in the same series (27). Baron (61) originally described an unusual form of osteomyelitis in 6 of 17 patients with bacillary angiomatosis. This infectious disease is caused by a rickettsia-like organism that is closely related to Rochalimaea quintana and has been identified by using a polymerase chain reaction that revealed a unique 165-gene sequence (27,61,81). Bacillary angiomatosis is marked by a cutaneous vascular lesion that occasionally infects the adjacent bone and creates osteomyelitis with osteolytic lesions (26,27). For more information on bacillary angiomatosis, please refer to Chapter 2.

In Vanarthos' series (63), a case of multifocal osteomyelitis caused by streptococcus group B was responsible for osteomyelitis with a few skip lesions in the distal tibia (Fig. 8). Mycobacterium haemophilium caused osteomyelitis in two cases reported by Gupta (70) and by Kristiansson (71) (Table 2). Salmonella osteomyelitis was noted in Spencer's (26) and Mastroianni's (68) reports. Isolated cases of bone infection due to gonococcus (72), cytomegalovirus (73), and candida albicans (74) osteomyelitis have been reported (Table 2).

The radiographic appearance of osteomyelitis in AIDS patients is similar to that of the general population. Bone scintigraphy, MRI and CT are very helpful for early diagnosis and imaging the extent of infection. The CT examination is advantageous for imaging of infection in flat bones of the pelvis and scapula (28).

Spondylitis in AIDS Patients

Among pyogenic causes, staph aureus remains the leading cause of septic spondylitis. The disc space is often involved and bony erosion of the adjacent end-plate is commonly the rule. Often, small or large epidural soft tissue involvement in the form of edema, inflammation or epidural abscess formation is noted (Figs. 9-11) (Table 3). In the case of M. tuberculosis, soft tissue abscess, when present, is seen anterior to the spine or iliopsoas area (cold abscess). In the

TABLE 2. OSTEOMYELITIS IN AIDS PATIENTS
"REVIEW OF LITERATURE"

Author	Ref. No.	No. of Cases	Microorganism
Baron	61	6	Bacillary angiomatosis
Steinbach	27	5	Staph aureus Nocardia asteroides Bacillary angiomatosis Unknown organism
Munoz-Fernandez	62	3	Bacteroide melaningenicus + Staph aureus Staph sanguis Staph aureus
Hughes	50	3	Salmonella enteritidis Histoplasma capsulatum Mycobacteria Kansasii
Vanarthos	63	2	Streptococcus Group B (multi-focal osteomyelitis) Other
Goh	64	1	Staph aureus
Zimmerman	65	1	Staph aureus
Jacobson	66	1	Staph aureus
Vail	67		
Mastroianni	68	1	Salmonella
Rubin	69	1	Torulopsis glabrata (hyoid bone)
Gupta	70	1	Mycobacteria haemophilum
Kristiansson	71	1	Mycobacteria haemophilum
Woods	72	1	Gonococcus
Berman	73	1	Cytomegalovirus (CMV)
Edelstein	74	1	Candida albicans

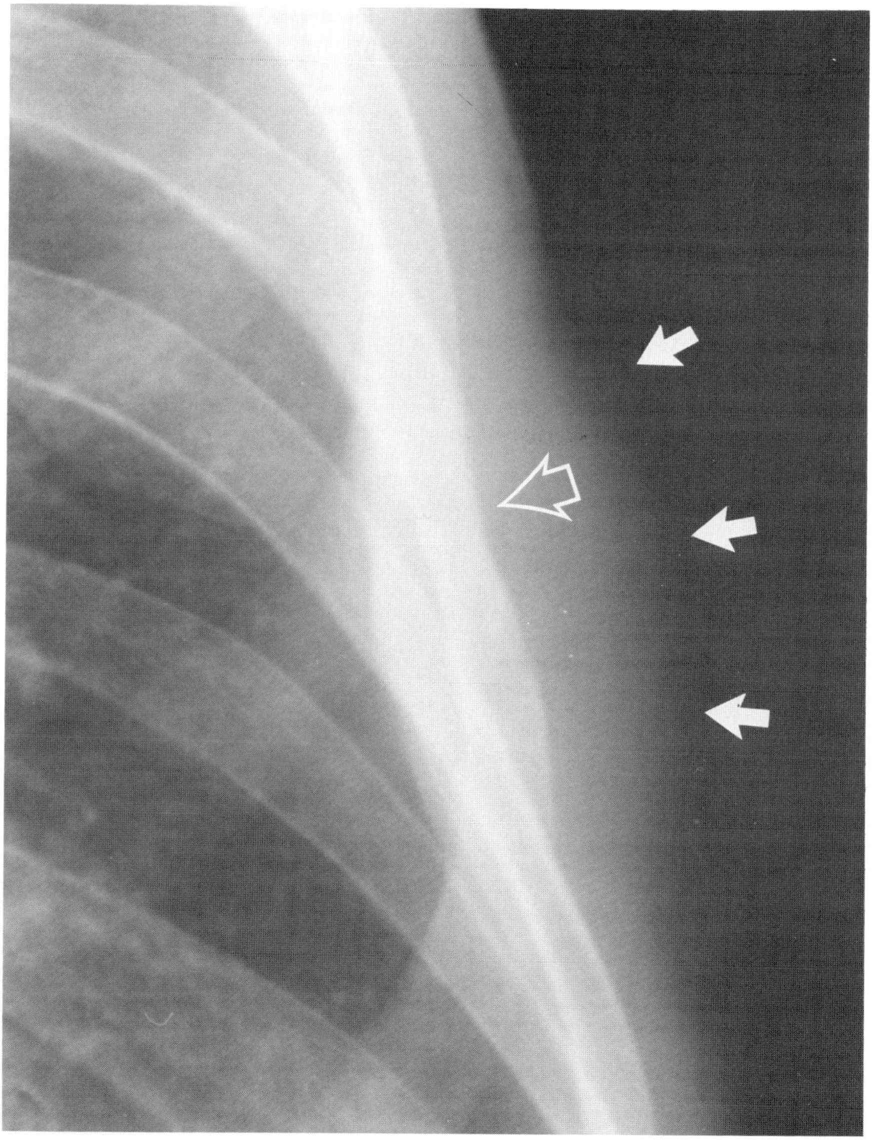

Figure 4-A

Multifocal osteomyelitis. 37-year-old HIV-positive female with history of candida esophagitis and left rib and left arm pain. The forearm and rib biopsies showed chronic infection and culture was negative. A and B. Plain radiographs of left ribs show soft tissue swelling (arrows) and bony erosion (open arrows) of sixth rib with pleural reaction.

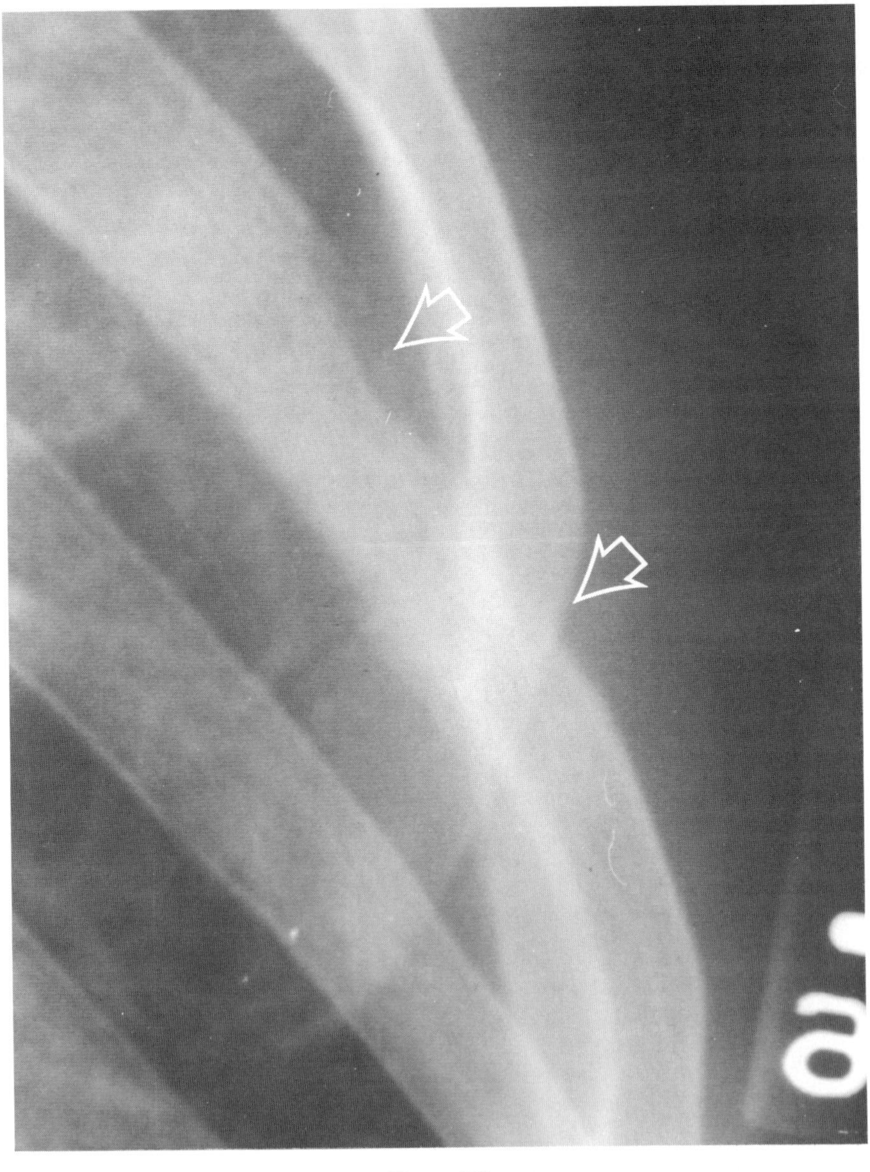

Figure 4-B

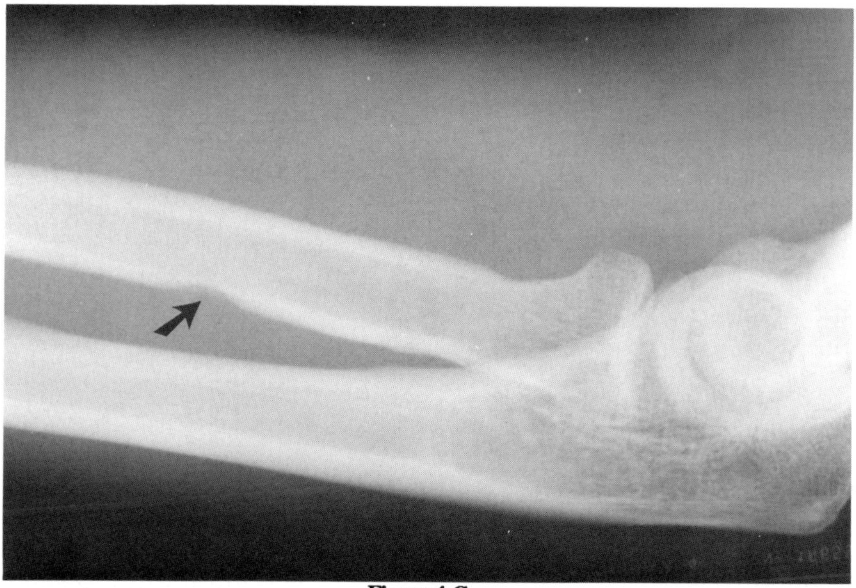

Figure 4-C

Lateral radiograph of the left forearm shows erosion of the posterior cortex of the proximal radial shaft (arrow).

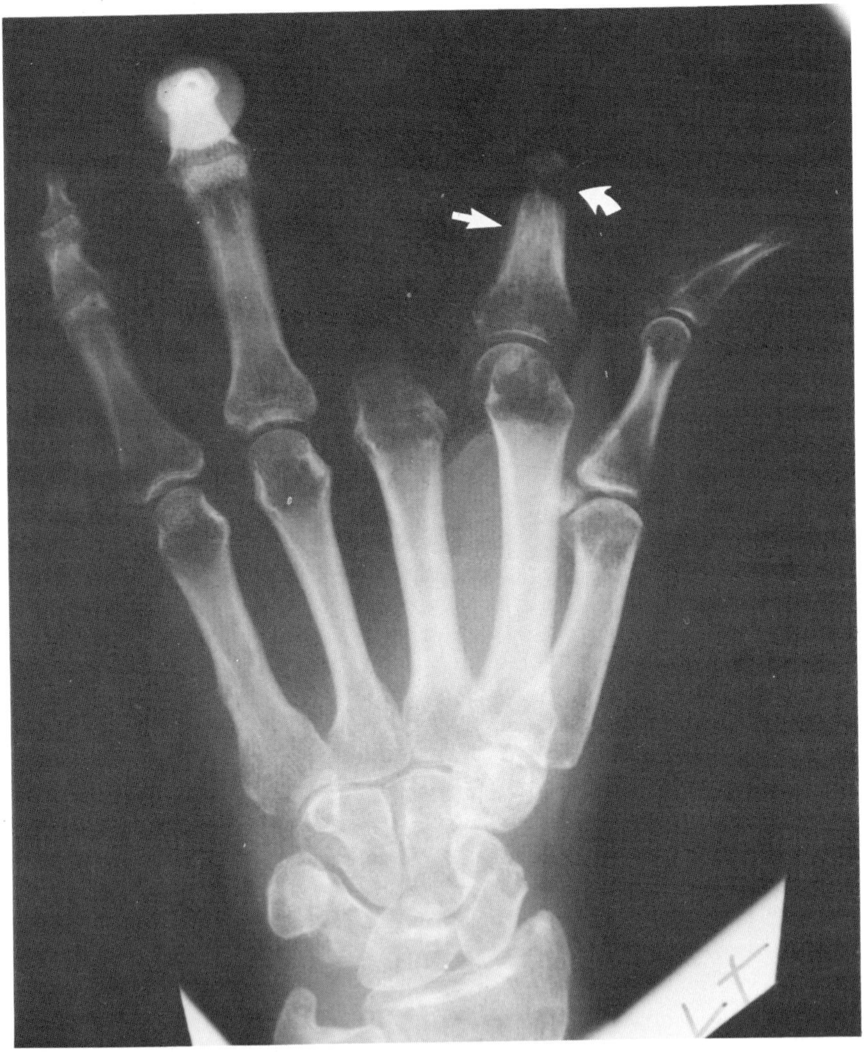

Figure 5

Repeated hand osteomyelitis. 31-year-old HIV-positive female. The patient had repeated episodes of osteomyelitis of the hand and had previous amputations of the second and third phalanges. Now there is recurrence of soft tissue and bone infection of the proximal phalanx of the index finger. AP view of the left hand shows osteopenia of the bones, flexion deformity and previous amputation. Note acute osteomyelitis of the partially amputated proximal phalanx of the index finger with bone erosion (curved arrow) and periosteal new bone formation (arrow).

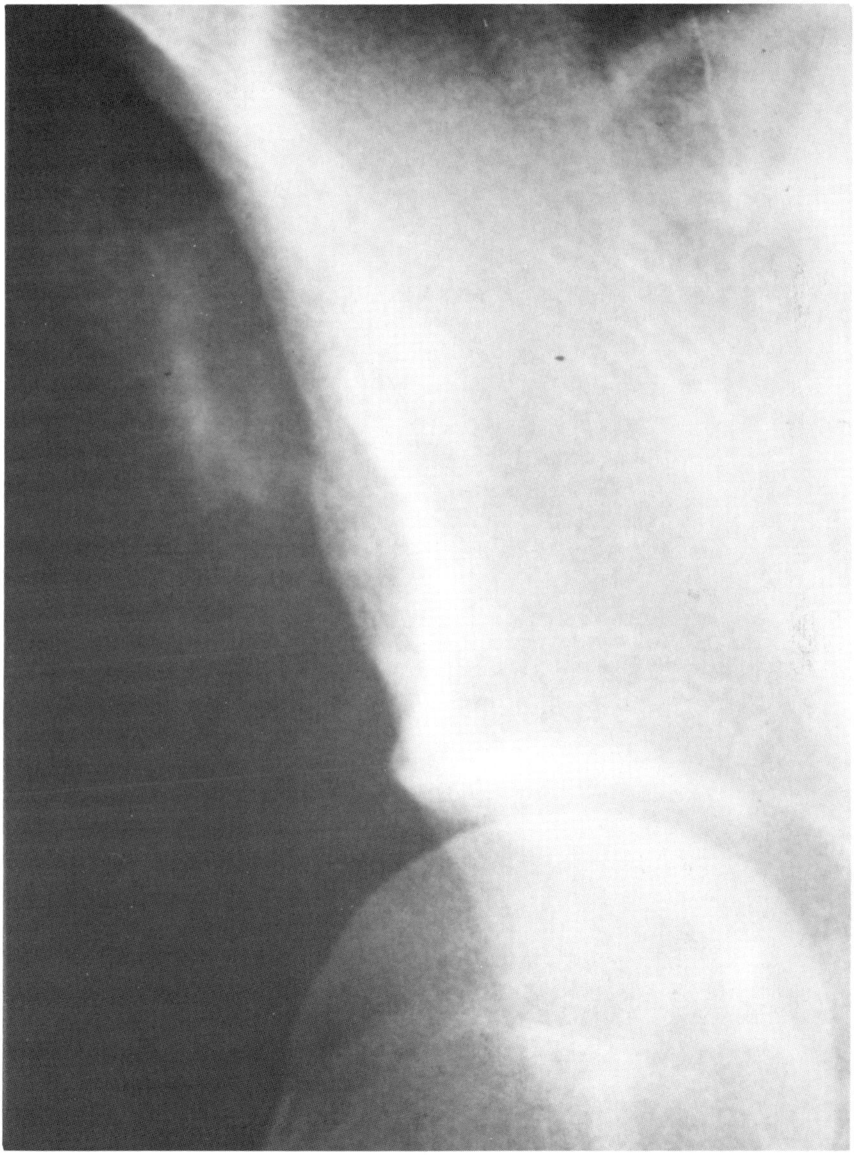

Figure 6-A

Osteomyelitis of iliac bone. 28-year-old HIV-positive black female with osteomyelitis of right iliac crest and heterotopic calcific changes. (From Vanarthos W: *RadioGraphics* 1992;12:731-749.) Plain radiograph shows heterotopic ossification with cortical erosion of the right iliac bone.

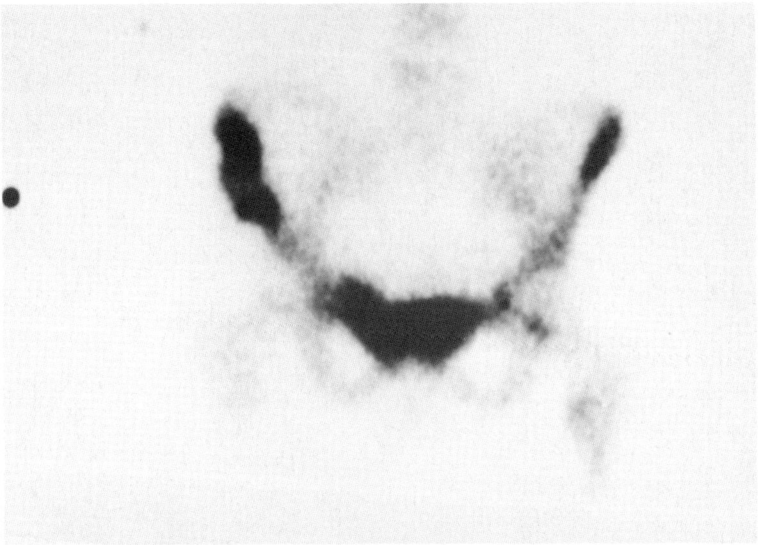

Figure 6-B

28-year-old HIV positive black female with osteomyelitis of right iliac crest and heterotopic calcific changes. Bone scan demonstrates increased activity in the right iliac bone.

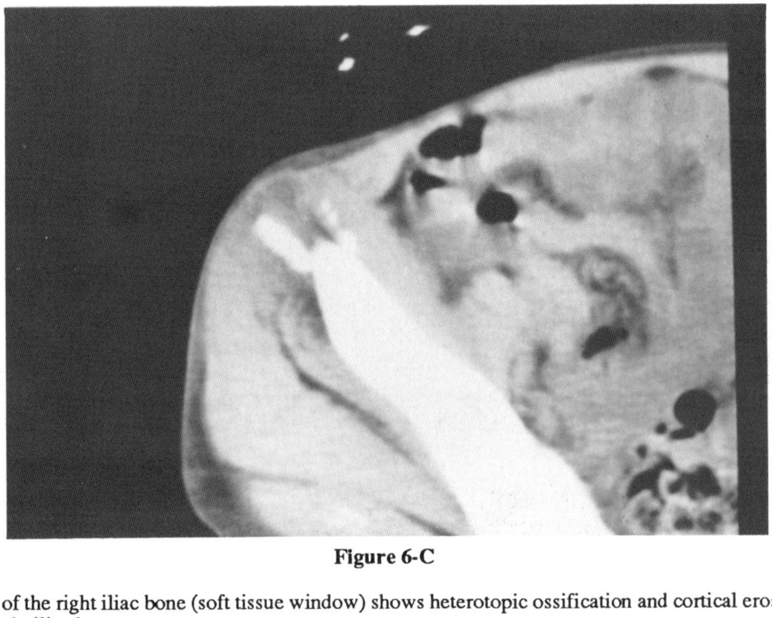

Figure 6-C

CT of the right iliac bone (soft tissue window) shows heterotopic ossification and cortical erosion of right iliac bone.

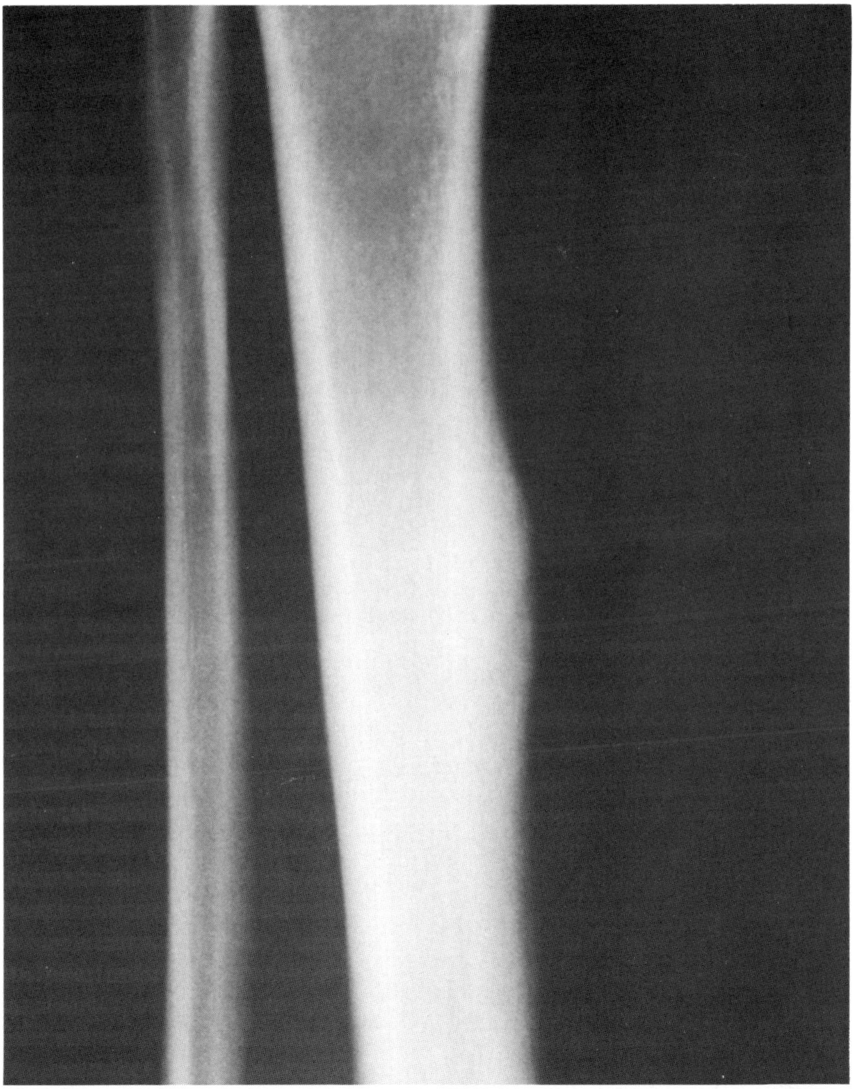

Figure 7-A

Osteomyelitis of tibia. 29-year-old HIV-positive female. Patient has a history of intravenous drug abuse and had several admissions for syphilis, gonorrhea and pelvic inflammatory disease. There is a leg ulcer and osteomyelitis of right tibia. Three-phase bone scan was positive at the tibial shaft and the culture grew pseudomonas aeroginosa and staph aureus. AP radiograph of the right tibia shows soft tissue ulcer of the anterior and medial tibial shaft. There is periostitis with cortical resorption and thickening.

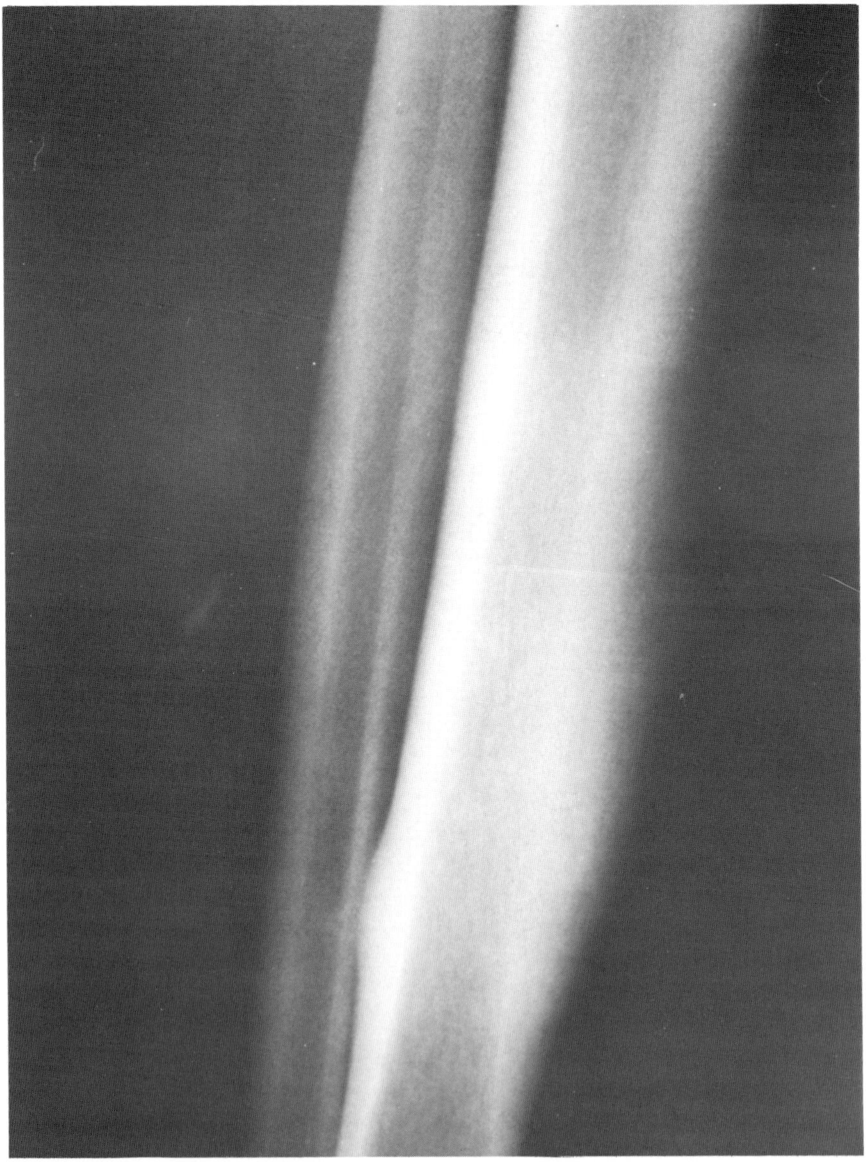

Figure 7-B

Lateral plain radiograph of the right tibia shows soft tissue ulcer of the anterior and medial tibial shaft. There is periostitis with cortical resorption and thickening.

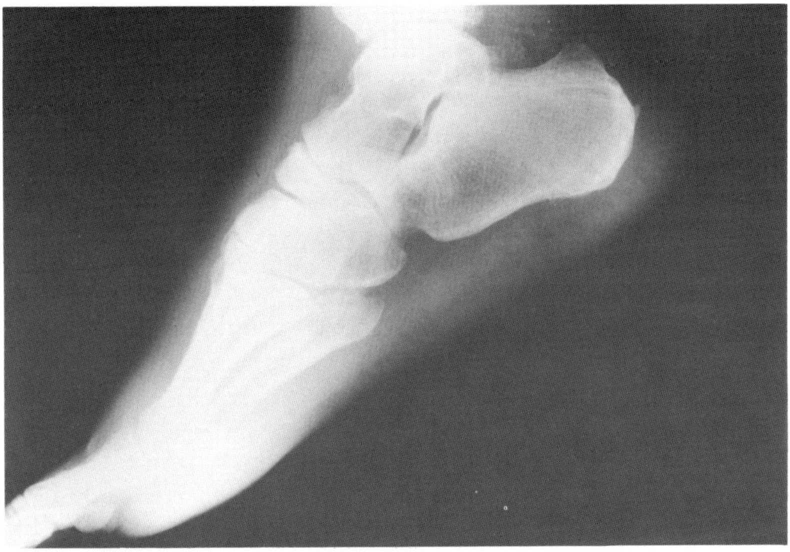

Figure 8-A

Multifocal osteomyelitis. 40-year-old HIV-positive Latino man with multifocal osteomyelitis of the right distal tibia due to group B streptococcus. (From Vanarthos W: RadioGraphics 1992;12:731-749.) Plain radiograph of the foot shows diffuse soft tissue swelling.

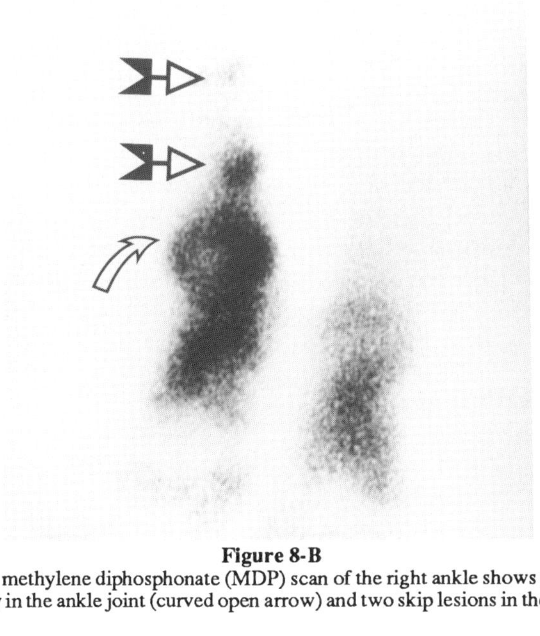

Figure 8-B

Anterior Tc-99m methylene diphosphonate (MDP) scan of the right ankle shows diffuse multifocal increased activity in the ankle joint (curved open arrow) and two skip lesions in the distal tibia (open arrows).

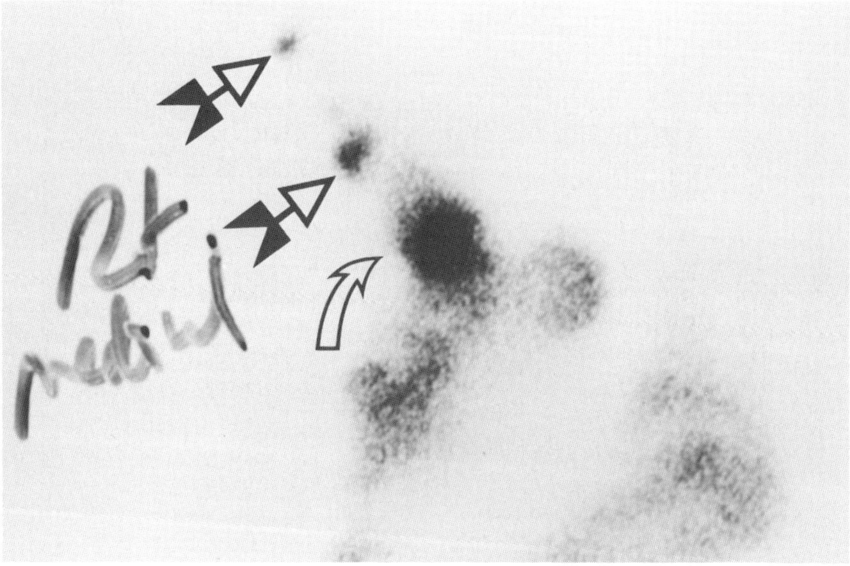

Figure 8-C
Medial Tc-99m methylene diphosphonate (MDP) scan of the right ankle shows diffuse multifocal increased activity in the ankle joint (curved open arrow) and two skip lesions in the distal tibia (open arrows).

large series of AIDS patients by Munoz-Fernandez (62), one case of M. tuberculosis was noted. Johnson (76) reported a 34-year-old man with HIV infection, M. tuberculosis, psoas abscess, and disseminated mycobacterium avium, and mycobacterium intracellulare infection. The abscess occurred 18 months after completion of a 12-month course of chemoprophylaxis with isoniazid that was given because of a positive reaction to tuberculin test (76).

Spinal tuberculosis is a relatively frequent finding in HIV-infected patients. Such patients are more likely to develop tuberculosis at extrapulmonary sites (82), a finding that is considered an AIDS-defining condition (76-83). For more information in regard to TB in AIDS patients, please refer to Chapter 3.

Pirofski (75) reported a case of an epidural abscess in an HIV-positive patient with a mixed staph aureus and cryptococcal infection. The diagnosis of cryptococcal meningitis and AIDS was made when cultures of CSF yielded cryptococcus neoformans and testing for human immunodeficiency virus (HIV) yielded a positive result (75). In Steinbach's series (27), one of 4 cases of spondylitis was caused by cryptococcus. In the same series, E. coli septicemia in an AIDS patient resulted in septic spondylitis with a large epidural abscess (Fig. 11) (Table 2). The third case of spondylitis was caused by staph aureus and

TABLE 3. SEPTIC SPONDYLITIS IN AIDS PATIENTS (REVIEW OF LITERATURE)

Author	Ref. No.	No. of Cases	Microorganism
Spinal Infection:			
Steinbach	27	4	Staph aureus E. coli Cryptococcus Unknown
Tehranzadeh	Current report		Candida tropicalis Pseudomonas
Munoz-Fernandez	62	1	Mycobacteria tuberculosis
Pirofski	75	1	Staph aureus and cryptococcus
Johnson	76	1	Mycobacteria avium & M. intracellulare
Boix	77	1	Candida albicans
Masters	78	1	Nocardia asteroides

the etiology for the fourth case was unknown. Boix (77) reported a spine infection with candida albicans in an AIDS patient. One of our two cases of spondylitis was noted in a 38-year-old woman with candida tropicalitis in the cervical spine, with a large anterior epidural abscess (Fig. 9). Our second case was a 31-year-old IV drug abuser with pseudomonas spondylitis (Fig. 10). MRI is helpful in imaging of spondylitis and discitis. With infection, a decreased signal intensity is noted in the disc space on T1WI (T1-weighted image), which increases on T2WI and is often associated with paraspinal or epidural inflammation, edema or abscess formation. The vertebral end-plates are also affected (28). The infection usually enhances following intravenous contrast administration.

Septic Arthritis

Arthralgias are a common complaint among HIV-positive patients. Although nonseptic arthritis such as rheumatoid arthritis and seronegative arthritides such as Reiter's and psoriasis are commonly reported in HIV-positive patients (These are discussed in Chapter 5.), septic arthritis is not as common except in HIV-positive patients who are also IV drug abusers (62). Despite this, the literature is replete with cases of septic arthritis in AIDS patients (27,50,62,63,74,84-108). It should be noted that the HIV virus has been isolated from synovial fluid of AIDS patients. This is not surprising since the virus is found in lymphocytes which are present in the synovium and synovial fluid (109). Staph aureus is again the most common cause of septic arthritis in AIDS patients (Table 4). In Munoz-Fernandez' series (62),10 of 17 cases of septic arthritis were due to staph aureus. Candida albicans was the second cause of septic arthritis in the same series and accounted for four cases (Table 4). All septic arthritis patients in this series were IV drug abusers (IVDA). Septic arthritis in IVDA has distinct clinical features such as the high prevalence in men, the young age of affected individuals, and the preferential localization to the fibrocartilaginous joints (62). In Monteagudo's series (85), three of six cases of septic arthritis in AIDS patients were due to staph aureus and one of the six cases was candida albicans.

Mycobacterium tuberculosis is the etiologic agent of septic arthritis in the four cases in Table 4 (27,63,85), and mycobacterium avium complex is responsible for two more cases of TB arthritis (91,99). Septic arthritis was caused by sporothrix Schenkii in two cases (90,92), gonococcus in two cases (95,96), and haemophilus influenza in two cases (103,104). Jarzem reported seven cases of septic arthritis in HIV-positive hemophiliacs (84). Septic arthritis in hemophiliacs most commonly involves the knee joint and is caused by staph aureus (86). Septic arthritis is becoming a more frequent complication of bacterial sepsis in HIV-infected hemophiliacs and is a new HIV-associated problem in this group. Thus, a hemophiliac who develops a hemarthrosis associated with fever, poor response to factor treatment, or multiple joint involvement should have joint

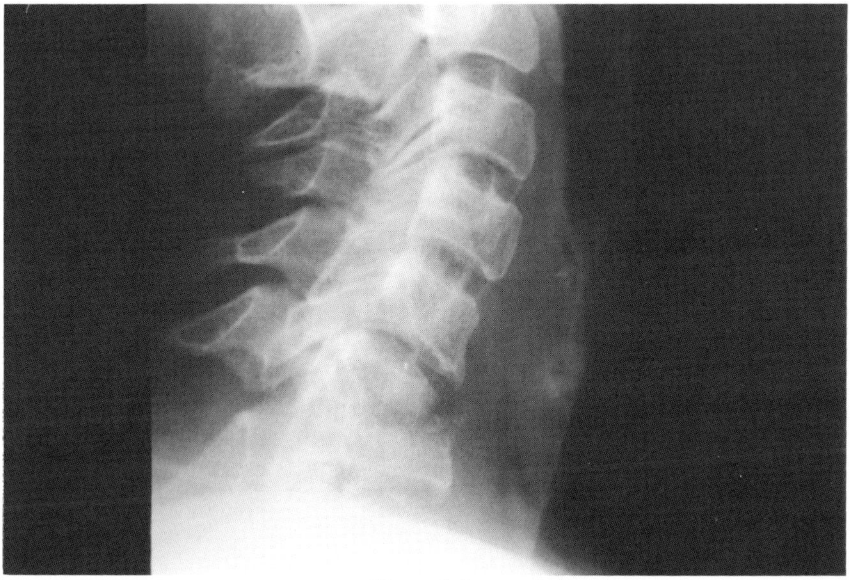

Figure 9-A

Cervical spondylitis and paravertebral abscess. 38-year-old HIV-positive female with candida tropicalis spondylitis at C6-C7 cervical spine. Lateral plain radiograph of cervical spine shows destructive changes and collapse of vertebral bodies of C6 and C7.

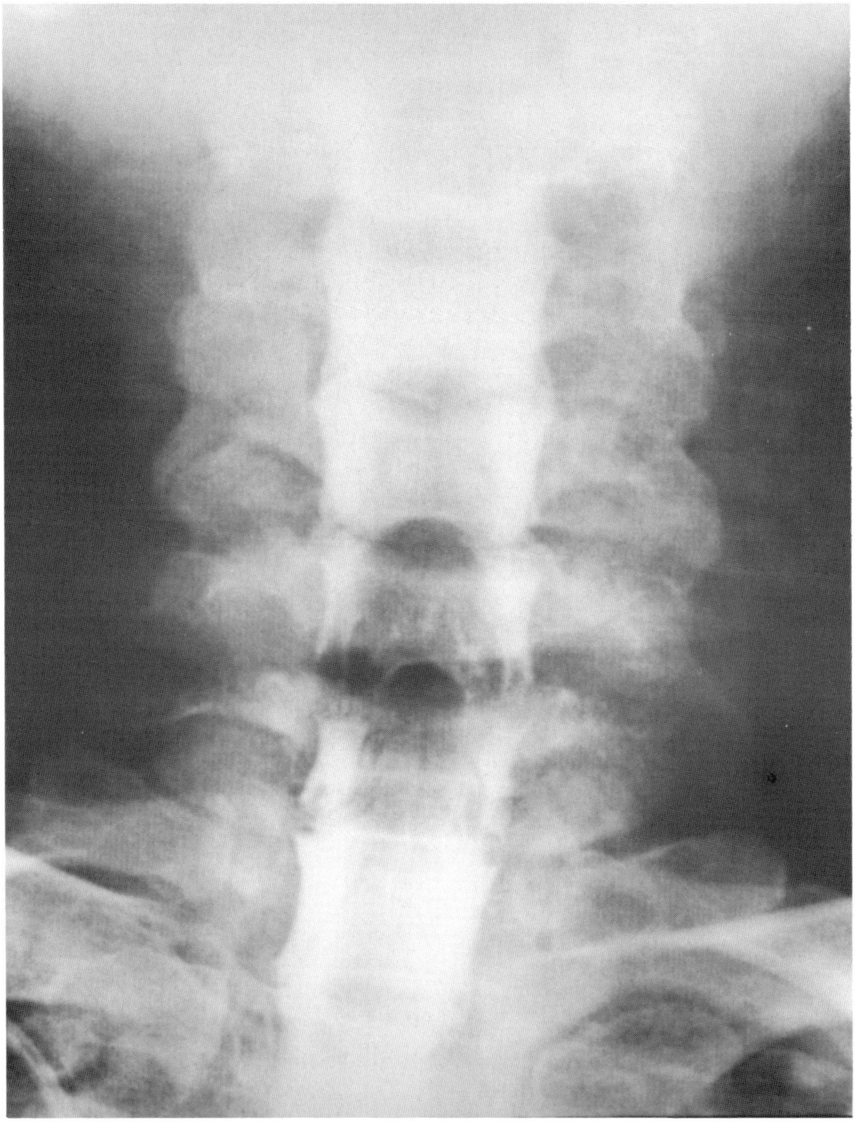

Figure 9-B
AP view of myelogram shows epidural defects at C6-7 bilaterally.

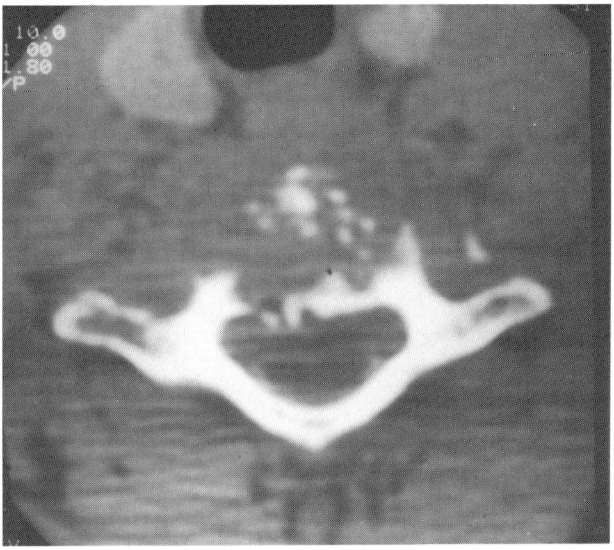

Figure 9-C
CT (bone window) of the cervical spine following myelogram at C6-7 shows destructive changes of vertebral end-plates.

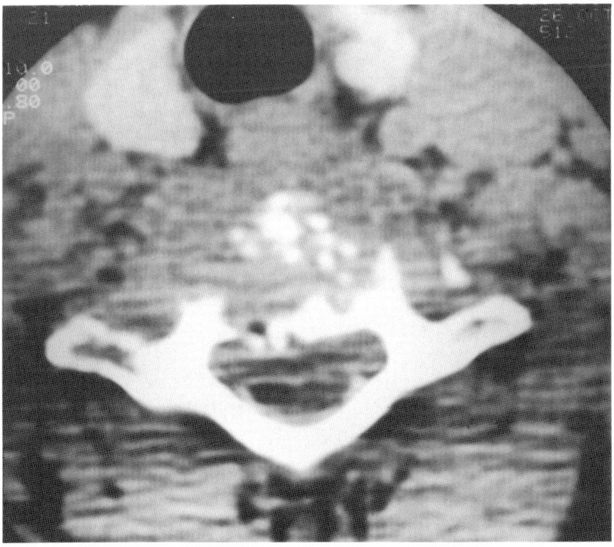

Figure 9-D
CT (soft tissue window) demonstrate anterior epidural and paravertebral soft tissue mass and inflammation.

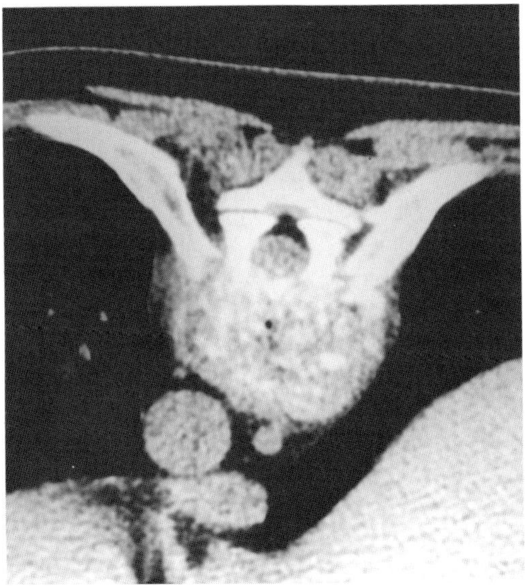

Figure 10-A

Thoracic spondylitis. 31-year-old HIV-positive female with history of intravenous drug abuse, with pseudomonas spondylitis. Prone CT of thoracic spine (bone window) at T7-8 shows destruction of vertebral end-plate and discitis.

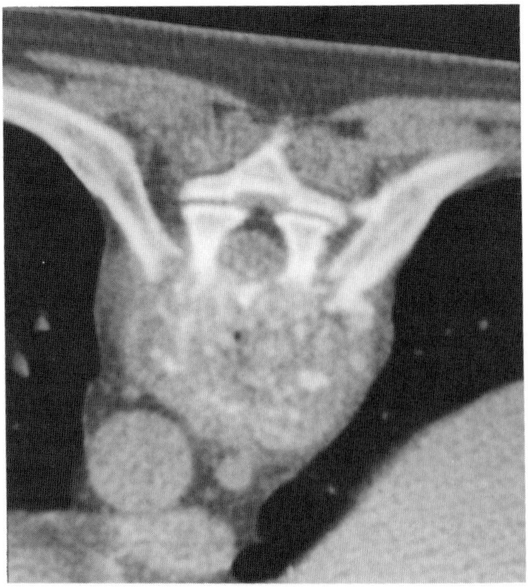

Figure 10-B

Soft tissue window of prone CT images shows paravertebral inflammation..

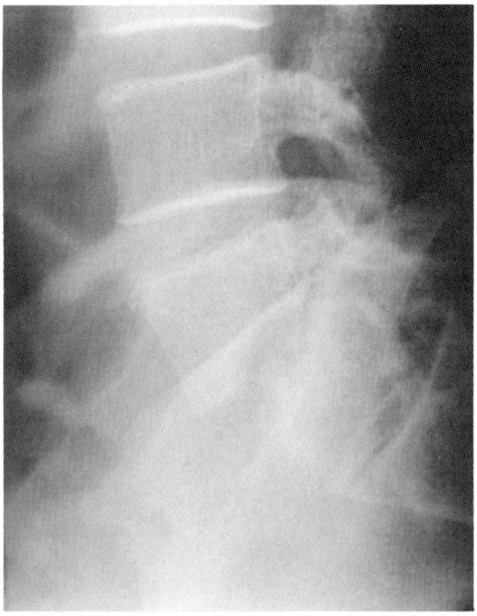

Figure 11-A

Lumbosacral spondylitis and paravertebral abscess. 45-year-old Latino man, HIV-positive, with history of E. coli septicemia a few months earlier, now presenting with septic spondylitis. Plain radiograph shows marked end-plate destruction of L5-S1 vertebra with grade I spondylolisthesis.

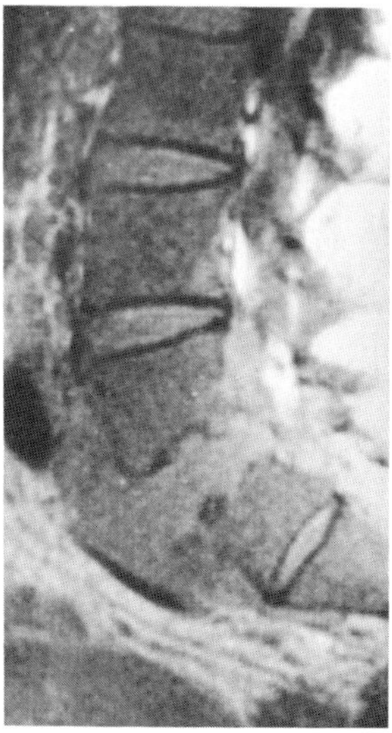

Figure 11-B

Sagittal T1-weighted image (TR 700/TE 20) shows end-plate erosion at L5-S1 with anterior paraspinal abscess extending to the disc and anterior epidural space.

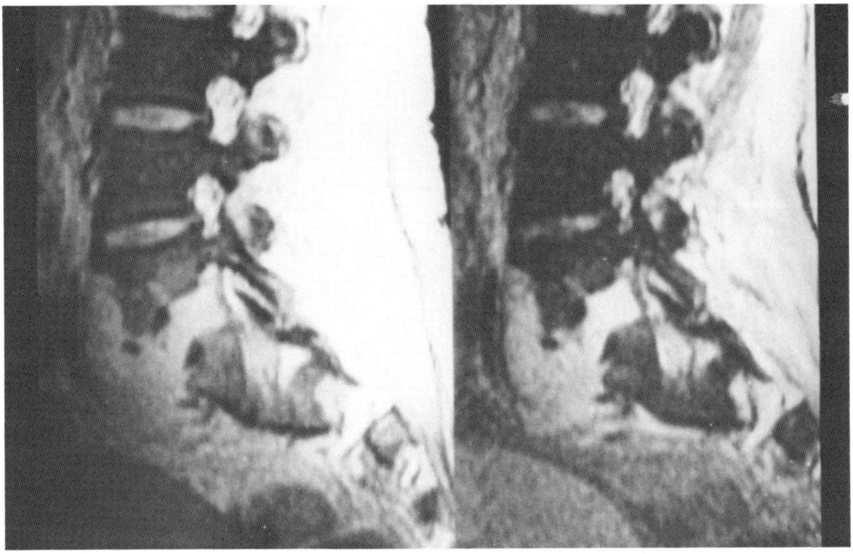

Figure 11-C

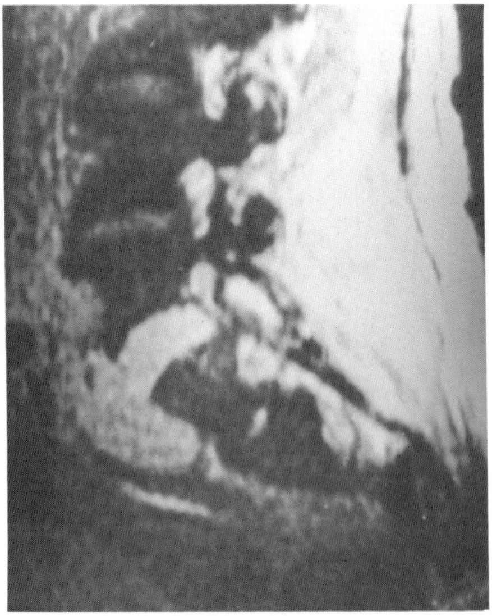

Figure 11-D

C. Sagittal proton density and T2-weighted images. D. T2-weighted image (TR2000/TE80) demonstrates large, high signal intensity paraspinal abscess.

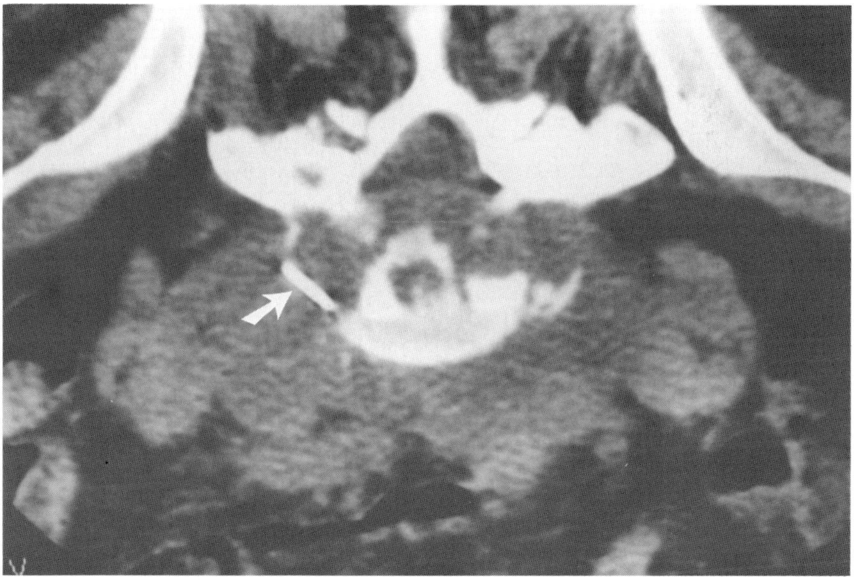

Figure 11-E
Prone CT (soft tissue window) of the pelvis at L5-S1 level shows bony destruction with large epidural and paraspinal abscess. Biopsy needle is also noted (arrow).

TABLE 4. SEPTIC ARTHRITIS IN AIDS PATIENTS (REVIEW OF LITERATURE)

Author	Ref.No.	No.of Cases	Microorganism
Munoz-Fernandez	62	17	Staph aureus
			Candida albicans
			Staph epidermidis
			Mucormycosis
			Bacteroides melaninogenicus
Jarzem	84	7	Septic arthritis cases in hemophiliacs
Hughes	50	7	Staph aureus
			Gram-negative bacilli
			Salmonella
			Histoplasma capsulatum
			Neisseria gonorrheae
			Pseudomonas sp.
Monteagudo	85	6	Staph aureus
			Candida albicans
			Mycobacteria tuberculosis
			Unknown
Steinbach	27	4	Pneumococcal arthritis
			Staph aureus
			Mycobacteria tuberculosis
Ragni	86	3	Staph aureus
			Streptococcus pneumoniae (polyarticular) (blood culture) hemophiliac
Pappo	87	3	Strep pneumoniae
			Staph aureus
Madariaga	88	1	Staph aureus

TABLE 4. SEPTIC ARTHRITIS IN AIDS PATIENTS
(Continued)

Author	Ref.No.	No.of Cases	Microorganism
Zimmerman	89	1	Staph aureus
Sokoloff	90	2	Staph aureus Sporothrix Schenkii
Vanarthos	63	2	Mycobacteria tuberculosis (sacroiliitis) Unknown
Vinetz	91	1	Mycobacteria avium complex
Lipstein-Kresch	92	1	Sporothrix Schenkii
Calabrese	93	1	Histoplasma capsulatum
Ricciardi	94	1	Cryptococcal
Strongin	95	1	Gonococcal (sternoclavicular)
Moyle	96	1	Gonococcal
Meyer	97	1	Candida albicans
Edelstein	74	1	Candida albicans
Hughes	98	1	Yersinia
Blumenthal	99	1	Mycobacteria avium complex
Luo	100	1	Salmonella
Mostaza	101	1	Mucormycosis
Burgoyne	102	1	Syphilitic polyarthritis
Lawrence	103	1	Haemophilus influenza
Fritz	104	1	Haemophilus influenza
Fenner	105	1	Chlamydia trachomatis
Glickel	106	1	--
Ike	107	1	Staph epidermis

aspiration and parenteral antibiotic therapy. Although this approach represents a departure from the standard avoidance of joint aspiration in these patients, aggressive management is necessary to avoid joint destruction, disability and spread to adjacent bones, which can be seen in this patient population (86,110).

Septic Bursitis

Infection in the subcutaneous bursa often localizes to the olecranon, prepatellar and, less frequently, subdeltoid regions. A history of recent trauma and occupational injury or puncture is frequently, although not invariably, present. Staphylococcus aureus is often the etiologic organism involved. Other less frequent agents include streptococcus pneumoniae, mycobacterium marinum, and sporothrix Schenkii. Hematogenous causes are uncommon (111).

Septic bursitis is a well-described entity in immunocompromised patients (50,112), including HIV-infected patients, alcoholics, and those who are on steroids. Buskila (112) has described two patients with staphylococcus aureus olecranon bursitis with evidence of HIV infection. Roschmann and Bell (113) have demonstrated that even though the presenting clinical features of septic bursitis in non-immunocompromised and immunocompromised patients are similar, immunocompromised patients must be treated with a significantly longer duration of therapy in order to guarantee a successful outcome.

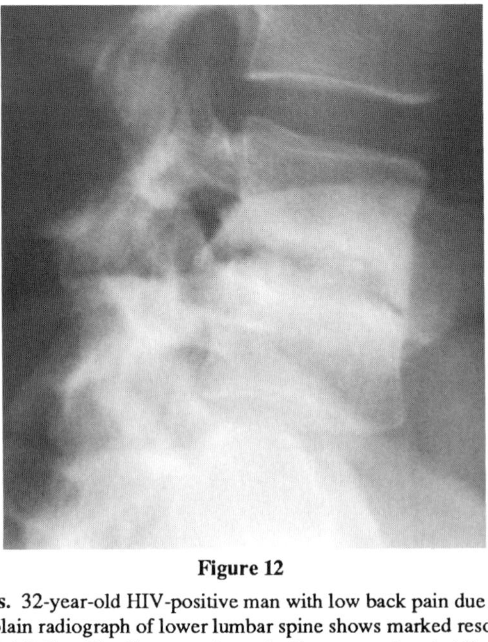

Figure 12

Lumbar spondylitis. 32-year-old HIV-positive man with low back pain due to cryptococcus spondylitis.Lateral plain radiograph of lower lumbar spine shows marked resorption and sclerosis of end-plates of L4-5 disc. The disc space is markedly narrowed and obliterated.

REFERENCES

1. CDC.: AIDS information cumulative cases documents nos. 320200,320201 and 320202, March 31,1993.
2. Curran JW, Morgan WM, Hardy AM, et al. The epidemiology of AIDS: current status and future prospects. *Science* 1985;229:1352-1357.
3. Piot P, Plummer FA, Mhalu FS, et al. AIDS: an international perspective. *Science* 1988;239:573-579.
4. Davenport C, Dillon WP, Sze G. Neuroradiology of the immunosuppressed state. *Rad Clin N Am* 1992;30(3):611-637.
5. Institute of Medicine Committee on a National Strategy for AIDS. Confronting AIDS: Directions for Public Health, Health Care, and Research. Washington, DC, *National Academy Press,* 1986.
6. Gottlieb MS, Schroff R, Schanker HM, Weisman JD, Fan PT, Wolf RA, Saxon A. Pneumocystis carinii pneumonia and mucosal candidiasis in previously healthy homosexual men. Evidence of a new acquired cellular immunodeficiency. *NEJM* 1981;305:1425-1431.
7. Barre-Sinoussi F, Chermann JC, Rey F, et al. Isolation of a T-lymphotropic retrovirus from a patient at risk for acquired immune deficiency syndrome (AIDS). *Science* 1983;220:868-871.
8. Popovic M, Sarngadharan MG, Read E, Gallo RC. Detection, isolation, and continuous production of cytopathic retroviruses (HTLV-III) from patients with AIDS and pre-AIDS. *Science* 1984;224:497-500.
9. Gallo RC, Salahuddin SZ, Popovic M, et al. Frequent detection and isolation of cytopathic retroviruses (HTLV-III) from patients with AIDS and at risk for AIDS. *Science* 1984;224:500-503.
10. Schupbach J, Popovic M, Gilden RU, Gonda MA, Sarngadharan MG, Gallo RC. Serological analysis of a subgroup of human T-lymphotropic retroviruses (HTL-VIII) associated with AIDS. *Science* 1984;224:503-505.
11. Epstein LG, Soudsmit J, Paul DA, Conner EM, Oleske JM HIV-specific antibodies and antigens in the cerebrospinal fluid of children with acquired immunodeficiency syndrome (AIDS) and AIDS-related complex (ARC). *Ann Neurol* 1986;20:433.
12. Buskila D, Gladman D. Musculoskeletal manifestations of infection with human immunodeficiency virus. *Rev Infect Dis* 1990;12(2):223-235.
13. Farizo KM, Buehler JW, Chamberland ME, et al. Spectrum of diseases in persons with human immunodeficiency virus infection in the United States. *JAMA* 1992; 267:1798-1805.
14. Rubin JT, Lotze MT. Immune function and dysfunction. A primer for the radiologist. *Rad Clin N Am* 1992;30(3):507-523.
15. McLoud TC, Naidich DP. Thoracic disease in the immunocompromised patient. *Rad Clin N Am* 1992;30(3):525-554.
16. Nelson JA, Wiley CA, Reynold-Kohler C, et al. Human immunodeficiency virus

detected in bowel epithelium from patients with gastrointestinal symptoms. *Lancet* 1988;1:259.

17. Jones B, Wall SD. Gastrointestinal disease in the immunocompromised host. *Rad Clin N Am* 1992;30(3):555-577.
18. Frager DH, Frager DJD, Brandt LJ, et al. Gastrointestinal complications of AIDS: radiologic features. *Radiology* 1986;158:597.
19. Levine MS, Woldenberg R, Herlinger H, et al. Opportunistic esophagitis in AIDS: radiographic diagnosis. *Radiology 1987;165:815.*
20. Levine MS, Macones PJ, Laufer I. Candida esophagitis: accuracy of radiographic diagnosis. *Radiology 1985;154:581.*
21. Balthazar EJ, Megibow AJ, Fazzini E, et al. Cytomegalovirus in AIDS: radiographic findings in 11 patients. *Radiology* 1985;155:585.
22. Jeffrey Jr RB. Abdominal imaging in the immunocompromised patient. *Rad Clin N Am 1992;30(3):579-596.*
23. de la Monte SM, Ho DD, Schooley RT, et al. Subacute encephalomyelitis of AIDS and its relation to HTLV-III infection. *Neurology* 1987;37:562-569.
24. Girolami V, Smith TW, Henin D, et al. Neuropathology of the acquired immunodeficiency syndrome. *Arch Pathol Lab* Med 1990;114:643-655.
25. Magid D, Fishman EK. Musculoskeletal infections in patients with AIDS: CT findings. *AJR* 1992;158:603-607.
26. Spencer M, Burgener FA, Hampton BA. Osteomyelitis in AIDS patient (abst.). *Radiology* 1991;181(P):155-156.
27. Steinbach LS, Tehranzadeh J, Fleckenstein JL, Vanarthos WJ, Pais MJ. Human immunodeficiency virus infection: musculoskeletal manifestations. *Radiology* 1993;186:833-838.
28. Tehranzadeh J, Wang F, Mesgarzadeh M Magnetic resonance imaging of osteomyelitis. *Crit Rev Diagn Imag* 1992;33(6):495-534.
29. Abrahamson SB, Odagnyk, Grieco AJ, Weissman G, Rosenstein A. Hyperalgesic pseudothrombophlebitis, a new syndrome in male homosexuals. *Am J Med* 1985; 78:317-320.
30. Schwartzman WA, Lambertus MW, Kennedy CA, Goetz MB. Staphylococcal pyomyositis in patient infected by the human immunodeficiency virus. *Am J Med* 1991;90(5):595-600.
31. Fleckenstein JL, Burns DK, Murphy FK, Jayson HT, Bonte FJ. Differential diagnosis of bacterial myositis in AIDS: evaluation with MR imaging. *Radiology* 1991;179:653-658.
32. Widrow C, Kellie S, Saltzman BR, Nadeson S, Mathur-Wagh U. Pyomyositis in HIV-infected patient. *Int Conf AIDS* 1990;6(2):367, (Abstract No. 2053).
33. Widrow CA, Kellie SM, Saltzman BR, Mathur-Wagh U. Pyomyositis in patients with human immunodeficiency virus: an unusual form of disseminated bacterial infection. *Am J Med* 1991;91(2):129-136.
34. Thomas R, French MA. Pyomyositis complicating the acquired immunodeficiency

syndrome: a report of two cases with coexistent neutropenia. *Med J Austral* 1991; 154(7):481-483.

35. Blumberg HM, Stephens DS. Pyomyositis and human immunodeficiency virus infection. *Southern Med J* 1990;83(9):1092-1095.
36. Balachandran, Thombish, McLean KA. Pyomyositis associated with AIDS (letter). *AIDS* 1990;4:471.
37. Wolf RF, Sprenger HG, Mooyuart EL, Tamsma JT, Kengan RA, Weits Jan. Nontropical pyomyositis as a cause of subacute syndrome. *Arthritis & Rheum* 1990;33:1728-1732.
38. Rodgers WB, Yodlowski ML, Mintzer CM. Pyomyositis in patients who have the human immunodeficiency virus. *J Bone Joint Surg* 1993;75-A(4):588-592.
39. Wu AW, Benirschke K, McCutchan JA. Rhabdomyolysis and staphylococcus aureus septicemia in a man with the acquired immunodeficiency syndrome. *West J Med* 1990;152(6):716-719.
40. Gardiner JS, Zank AM, Minnefor AB, Boyd LC, Avella DG, McInerney VK. Pyomyositis in an HIV-positive premature infant: case report and review of the literature. *J Pediatr Orthop* 1990;10(6):791-793.
41. Wrzolek MA, Sher JH, Kozlowski PB, Rao C. Skeletal muscle pathology in AIDS: an autopsy study. *Muscle Nerve* 1990;13(6):508-515.
42. Pouchot J, Vinceneux P, Barge, Laparre F, BoussouGaut Y, Michon C. Tuberculous polymyositis in HIV infection (letter). *Am J Med* 1990;89(2):250-251.
43. Gaut P, Wong PK, Meyer RD. Pyomyositis in a patient with the acquired immunodeficiency syndrome. *Arch Int Med* 1988;148(7):1608-1610.
44. Vartian C, Septimus EJ. Pyomyositis in an intravenous drug user with human immunodeficiency virus (letter). *Arch Int Med* 1988;148(12):2689.
45. Raphael SA, Wolfson BJ, Parker P, Lischner HW, Faerber EN. Pyomyositis in a child with acquired immunodeficiency syndrome: patient report and brief review. *Am J Dis Child* 1989;143(7):779-781.
46. Victor G, Branley J, Opal SM, Meyer KH. Pyomyositis in a patient with acquired immunodeficiency syndrome (letter). *Arch Int Med* 1989;149(3):705-709.
47. Elsing C, Erckenbrecht JF, Borchard F, Strohmeyer G. Tropical diseases of HIV patients in non-endemic countries: a case of visceral Leishmaniasis and a case of tropical pyomyositis. Int Conf on AIDS 1989;5:238 (Abstract No. MBP 100).
48. Belec L, Costanzo B, Georges AJ, Gherardi R. HIV infection in African patient with tropical pyomyositis (letter). *AIDS* 1991;5(2):234.
49. Watts RA, Hoffbrand BI, Paton DF, Davis JC. Pyomyositis associated with human immunodeficiency virus infection. *Brit Med J* (Clin Res Ed) 1987;13:294(6586): 1524-1525.
50. Hughes RA, Row IF, Shanson D, Keat AC. Septic bone, joint and muscle lesions associated with human immunodeficiency virus infection. *Brit J Rheumatol* 1992; 31(6):381-388.

51. Ras GJ, Anderson R, Lecatsas G, Sher R. Acquired neutrophil dysfunction in male homosexuals with the acquired immunodeficiency syndrome. *S Afr Med J* 1984; 65:873-874.
52. Ras GJ, Eftychis HA, Anderson R, van der Walt I. Mononuclear and polymorphonuclear leukocyte dysfunction in male homosexuals with the acquired immunodeficiency syndrome (AIDS). *S Afr Med J* 1984;66:806-809.
53. Valone FH, Payan DG, Abrams DI, Goetzl EJ. Defective polymorphonuclear leukocyte chemotaxis in homosexual men with persistent lymph node syndrome. *J Infect Dis* 1984;150:267-271.
54. Niclsen H, Kharazmi A, Faber V. Blood monocyte and neutrophil functions in the acquired immune deficiency syndrome. *Scand I Immunol* 1986;24:291-296.
55. Lazzarin A, Uberti Foppa C, Galli M, et al. Impairment of polymorphonuclear leukocyte function in patients with acquired immunodeficiency syndrome and with lymphadenopathy syndrome. *Clin Exp Immunol* 1986;65:105-111.
56. Ellis M, Gupta S, Galant S, et al. Impaired neutrophil function in patients with AIDS or AIDS-related complex: a comprehensive evaluation. *J Infect Dis* 1988;158:1268-1276.
57. Martin LS, Spira TJ, Orloff SL, Holman RC. Comparison of methods for assessing chemotaxis of monocytes and polymorphonuclear leukocytes isolated from patients with AIDS or AIDS-related conditions. *J Leukoc Biol* 1988;44:361-366.
58. Roilides E, Mertins S, Eddy J, et al. Impairment of polymorphonucleocyte (PMN) chemotactic and bactericidal function in HIV-infected children (Abstract Th.B.P.89). *Fifth International Conference on AIDS,* Montreal, Canada, 1989:430.
59. Murphy M, Buckley M, Corr J, Vinayagamoorthy S, Grainger R, Mulcahy FM. Founier's gangrene of scrotum in a patient with AIDS. *Genitourin Med* 1991;67: 339-341.
60. Chiedozi LC. Pyomyositis: review of 205 cases in 112 patients. *Am J Surg* 1979; 137:255-259
61. Baron AL, Steinbach LS, LeBoit PE, Mills CM, Gee JH, Berger TG. Osteolytic lesions and bacillary angiomatosis in HIV infection: radiologic differentiation from AIDS-related Kaposi sarcoma. *Radiology* 1990;177:77-81.
62. Munoz-Fernandez S, Auiralte J, del Arco A, Balsa A, Cardenal A, Pena JM, Vazquez n Gilon Banos J. Osteoarticular infection associated with the human immunodeficiency virus. *Clin Exper Rheumatol* 1991;9(5):489-493.
63. Vanarthos W, Ganz WI, Vanarthos JC, Serafini AN, Tehranzadeh J. Diagnostic uses of nuclear medicine in AIDS. *RadioGraphics* 1992;12:731-749.
64. Goh BT, Jawad AS, Chapman D, Winceslaus SJ, Froster GE, Perry JD. Osteomyelitis presenting as a swollen elbow in a patient with the acquired immune deficiency syndrome. *Ann Rheum Dis* 1988;47(8):695-696.
65. Zimmerman B 3rd, Erickson AD, Milkolich DJ. Septic acromioclavicular arthritis and osteomyelitis in a patient with acquired immunodeficiency syndrome. *Arth & Rheum* 1989;32(9):1175-1178.
66. Jacobson MA, Gellerman H, Chambers H. Staphylococcus aureus bacteremia and

recurrent staphylococcal infection in patients with acquired immunodeficiency syndrome and AIDS-related complex. *Am J Med* 1988;85:172-176.

67. Vail TP, Urbaniak JR. Hematogenous patellar osteomyelitis with human immunodeficiency virus. *Orthop Rev* 1991;20(9):788-790.
68. Mastroianni CM, Vullo V, Delia S. Cranial salmonella abscess with parietal bone osteomyelitis in an HIV-infected patient (letter). *AIDS* 1992;6(7):749-750.
69. Rubin MM, Sanfilippo RJ. Osteomyelitis of the hyoid caused by torulopsis glabrata in a patient with acquired immunodeficiency syndrome. *J Oral Maxillofac Surg* 1990;48(11):1217-1219.
70. Gupta I, Kocher J, Miller AJ, Weisholtz SJ, Perz J, Scully M. Mycobacterium haemophilum osteomyelitis in an AIDS patient. *New Jersey Medicine* 1992;89(3): 201-202.
71. Kristiansson M, Bieluch VM, Bveff PD. Mycobacterium haemophilum infection in immunocompromised patients: case report and review of the literature. *Rev Infect Dis* 1991;13(5):906-910.
72. Woods SM, Gernaat HB. Gonococcal osteomyelitis in a Zambian patient with AIDS. *Tropical Doctor* 1992;22(1):47-48.
73. Berman S, Jensen J. Cytomegalovirus-induced osteomyelitis in a patient with the acquired immunodeficiency syndrome. *South Med J* 1990;83(10):1231-1232.
74. Edelstein H, McCabe R. Candida albicans, septic arthritis and osteomyelitis of the sternoclavicular joint in a patient with human immunodeficiency virus infection. *J Rheumatol* 1991;18(1):110-111.
75. Pirofski L, Casadevall A. Mixed staphylococcal and cryptococcal epidural abscess in a patient with AIDS (letter, comment). *Rev Infect Dis* 1990;12(5):964-965.
76. Johnson SC, Stamm CP, Hicks CB. Tuberculous psoas muscle abscess following chemoprophylaxis with Isoniazid in a patient with human immunodeficiency virus infection. *Rev Infect Dis* 1990;12(5):754-756.
77. Boix V, Tovar J, Martin-Hidalgo A. Candida spondylodiscitis: chronic illness due to heroin analgesia in an HIV-positive person (letter). *J Rheumatol* 1990;17(4): 563-565.
78. Masters DL, Lentiro JR. Cervical osteomyelitis related to nocardia asteroides. *J Infect Dis* 1984;149:824-825.
79. Sabbagh M, Meyer O, DeBandt M, Salomon-Caron D, Perrone C, Rosenbaum W, Tremoliere F, Kahn MF. Bone manifestations associated with acquired immuno deficiency syndrome (AIDS). *Annales de Medecine Interne* 1992;143(1):50-56.
80. Roder W, Muller H, Muller WE, Merz H. HIV infection in human bone. *J Bone Joint Surg, British Volume* 1992;74(2):179-180.
81. Relman DA, Lontit JS, Schmidt TM, Falkow S, Tompkins LS. The agent of bacillary angiomatosis: an approach to the identification of uncultured pathogenes. *NEJM* 1990;323:1573-1580.
82. Sunderam G, McDonald RJ, Maniatis T, Oleske J, Kapila R, Reichman LB.

Tuberculosis as a manifestation of the acquired immunodeficiency syndrome (AIDS). *JAMA* 1986;256:362-366.

83. Centers for Disease Control. Revision of the CDC surveillance case definition for acquired immunodeficiency syndrome. *MMWR* 1987;36(suppl 1):1S-15S.
84. Jarzem P, Tsoukas C, Burke D, Strawczynski H, Growe G, Poon MC. Hemophilia, septic arthritis and human immunodeficiency virus. Int Conf on AIDS 1989;5:416 (Abstract No. Th.B.P.7).
85. Monteagudo I, Rivera J, Lopez-Longo J, Cosin J, Garcia-Monforte A, Carreno L. AIDS and rheumatic manifestations in patients addicted to drugs: an analysis of 106 cases. *J of Rheumatol* 1991;18(7):1038-1041.
86. Ragni MV, Haneley EN. Septic arthritis in a hemophiliac patient and infection with human immunodeficiency virus (HIV) (letter). *Ann Int Med* 1989;15:110(2): 168-169.
87. Pappo AS, Buchanan GR, Johnson RA. Septic arthritis in children with hemophilia. *Am J Dis Child* 1989;143:1226-1228.
88. Madariaga L, Aramburu JM, Suarez MB, Gorodo JM, Anton I, Lardelli P, Campelo C, Cisterna R. Presence of HIV antigen P24 in the synovial fluid of a patient without antigenemia suffering from staphylococcal arthritis (letter). *AIDS* 1991;5(3):337-338.
89. Zimmerman B III, Erickson AD, Mikolich DJ. Septic acromioclavicular arthritis and osteomyelitis in a patient with acquired immunodeficiency syndrome. *Arthr &Rheum* 1989;32(9):1175-1178.
90. Sokoloff L. A prospective necropsy study of arthritis in acquired immunodeficiency syndrome. *Arch Pathol Lab Med* 1990;114(10):1035-1037.
91. Vinetz JM, Rickman LS. Chronic arthritis due to mycobacterium avium complex infection in a patient with the acquired immunodeficiency syndrome. *Arthr & Rheum* 1991;34(10):1339-1340.
92. Lipstein-Kresch E, Isenberg HD, Singer C, Cooke 0, Greenwald RA. Disseminated sporothrix Schenckii infection with arthritis in a patient with acquired immunodeficiency syndrome. *J Rheumatol* 1985;12:805-808.
93. Calabrese LH. The rheumatic manifestations of infection with the human immunodeficiency virus. *Semin Arth Rheum* 1989;18:225-239.
94. Ricciardi DD, Sepkowitz DV, Berkowitz LB, Bienenstock H, Maslow M. Cryptococcal arthritis in a patient with acquired immune deficiency syndrome. Case report and review of the literature. *J Rheumatol* 1986;13(2):455-458.
95. Strongin IS, Kale SA, Raymond MK, Luskin RL, Weisberg GW, Jacobs JJ. An unusual presentation of gonococcal arthritis in an HIV-positive patient. *Ann Rheumat Dis* 1991;50(8):572-573.
96. Moyle G, Barthon SE, Midgley J, Powe IF, Keat AC, Lawrence AG. Gonococcal arthritis caused by anxotype P in a man with (HIV) infection. *Genitourin Med 1990;* 66(2):91-92.
97. Meyer RD, Gaut PL. Candidal pyarthritis in an AIDS patient. *Scand J Infect Dis* 1990;22(5):607-610.

98. Hughes RA, Keat AC. Yersinia reactive arthritis and human immunodeficiency virus infection (letter). *Arthr &Rheum* 1990;33(5):758-759.
99. Blumenthal DR, Zucker JR, Hawkins CC. Mycobacterium avium complex-induced septic arthritis and osteomyelitis in a patient with the acquired immunodeficiency syndrome (letter). *Arthr & Rheum* 1990 May;33(5):757-758.
100. Luo NP, Perera CU, Zumla A. Salmonella septic arthritis. *J of Infect* 1991;23(1): 101.
101. Mostaza JM, Barbado FJ, Fernandez-Montin J, Peña-Yañez J, Vasquez-Rodriguez JJ. Cutaneoarticular mucormycosis due to cunning hamella bertholletiae in a patient with AIDS. *Rev Infect Dis* 1989;11(2):316-318.
102. Burgoyne M, Agudelo C, Pisko E. Chronic syphilitic polyarthritis mimicking systemic lupus erythematosus/rheumatoid arthritis as the initial presentation of human immunodeficiency virus infection. *J Rheumatol* 1992;19(2):313-315.
103. Lawrence JM III, Osborn TG, Paro R, Eaton C, Hyers TM, Moore TL. Septic arthritis caused by hemophilus influenza type B in a patient with HIV infection. *J of Rheumatol 1991;18(11):1772-1773.*
104. Fritz P, Bardin T, Vittecog D. Septic arthritis due to haemophilus influenza in a patient with HIV infection (letter). *Clin Exper Rheumatol* 1991;9(1):91-93.
105. Fenner T, Fenner I, Hoffman A, Schrappe M, Albig S, Rascot H, Schmitz H. Detection of chlamydia trachomatis in synovial fluid of human immunodeficiency virus type 1 infected patients with acute arthritis using polymerase chain reaction (PCR). *International Conference on AIDS* 1992;8(3):78, (Abstract No. Pub. 7178).
106. Glickel SZ. Hand infections in patients with acquired immunodeficiency syndrome. *J Hand Surg[Am]* 1988;13:770-775.
107. Ike RW. Arthroscopy in septic arthritis of the knee: spectrum of applications. *Arthritis & Rheum* 1990;33(Suppl):887.
108. Bleasel JF, York JR, Rickand KA. Septic arthritis in human immunodeficiency virus-infected haemophiliacs (letter). *Brit J Rheumatol* 1990;29(6):494-496.
109. Stein M, Davis P. HIV and arthritis: causal or casual acquaintances? *J of Rheumatol* 1989;16(10):1287-1289.
110. Goldenberg DL, Reed JI. Bacterial arthritis. *NEJM* 1985;312:764-771.
111. Resnick D, Niwayama G (eds). *Diagnosis of Bone and Joint Disorders.* Philadelphia: W.B. Saunders Co., 1988.
112. Buskila D, Tenenbaum J. Septic bursitis in human immunodeficiency virus infection. *J of Rheumatol* 1989;16(10):1374-1376.
113. Roschmann RA, Bell CL. Septic bursitis in immunocompromised patients. *Am J Med* 1987;83: 661-665.

CHAPTER 2:

BACILLARY ANGIOMATOSIS

Lynne S. Steinbach, M.D.

BACKGROUND

Bacillary angiomatosis is a recently described disorder that results from infection with organisms from the rickettsiaceae family, Rochalimaea henselae and Rochalimaea quintana — which are also suspected agents for cat-scratch disease and trench fever, respectively (1-5). This illness occurs predominantly in patients infected with human immunodeficiency virus (HIV) and typically produces angiomatous cutaneous lesions that can be accompanied by bacteremia, adenitis, aseptic meningitis, intracerebral mass lesions, osseous lesions, and peliosis hepatis.

Bacillary angiomatosis has been seen in patients with HIV infection and in those with drug-induced immune suppression. The diagnosis of cutaneous bacillary angiomatosis and parenchymal bacillary peliosis should also be included in immunocompetent patients, as it is being increasingly reported in people with normal cellular and humoral immunity who have no evidence of HIV infection, using a combination of sensitive HIV antibody and antigen assays as well as viral culture and polymerase chain-reaction techniques (4,6,7,8). Bacillary splenitis can be seen in the absence of peliosis and appears to be another manifestation of R. henselae infection (7). The organism can also produce bacteremia in immunocompromised and immunocompetent hosts (3,8). It has been associated with aseptic meningitis and, like R. quintana and Bartonella spp., can be seen with relapsing disease and with persistent bacteremia in the absence of symptoms (9-14).

Characteristics of the Bacterial Agent

Until recently, it was difficult to isolate and culture the organism that causes bacillary angiomatosis. The pathogens, R. henselae and R. quintana, which have been identified as the etiologic agents for bacillary angiomatosis, have now been isolated by two methods. Relman, et al. (15) amplified the 16S ribosomal RNA gene from bacillary angiomatosis lesions using a polymerase chain reaction, which was found to be similar to that of R. quintana, the organism that causes trench fever. The organism was also isolated in primary culture of blood after lysis-centrifugation in five patients with fever (4,8). Koehler, et al. (1) cultured organisms from cutaneous bacillary angiomatosis lesions of four patients and analysis of the amplified 16S r DNA sequence indicated that the organism was R. quintana in three patients and R. henselae in one.

Pleomorphic bacilli may be visualized on Warthin-Starry silver-stained tissue specimens (Fig. 1) and trilaminar-walled organisms are identified by electron microscopy. Slow growth, X-factor dependence, specific membrane fatty acid analysis by gas chromatography, negative oxidase, catalase and urease, as well as appearance as a pleomorphic, curved gram-negative rod on gram stain help to identify R. henselae. It can be difficult to isolate R. henselae from tissue in the laboratory. Special preparation includes inoculation of the sample directly onto a fresh blood or chocolate agar plate in increased CO_2. The plates should be kept for as long as six weeks and dessication should be avoided by storing them in a gas-permeable, moisture-retaining envelope (5).

Cat-scratch disease (CSD) is a closely related disorder which was first recognized in the 1930s but was not reported until 1950. Until 1983, cat-scratch disease was diagnosed solely on the basis of clinical criteria. Wear and coworkers (16) identified bacilli from a lymph node of a patient with CSD in 1983, establishing it as an infectious disorder. There is increasing proof that CSD is also caused by Rochalimaea infection (17). R. henselae has been isolated from the blood of a Rochalimaea-seropositive cat, which also supports this assumption (18). R. henselae is characterized as oxidase-negative and X-factor-dependent and in analysis has a characteristic pattern of whole-cell fatty acids. This differs from the gram-negative rod, Afipia felis, which had previously been associated with cat-scratch disease. Afipia felis is oxidase-positive and has a different whole-cell fatty acid content (4,5,19). In fact, there is evidence that A. felis has only rarely been isolated from patients with CSD and that A. felis-specific antibodies are lacking in most persons with suspected cat-scratch disease. Nearly 90% of persons with suspected CSD have serologic evidence of Rochalimaea infection (17).

Clinical Manifestations

Bacillary angiomatosis is characterized by a distinct vascular proliferation in the skin, viscera, lymph nodes, brain, and bone (1,20,21). It has been recognized increasingly since the onset of the AIDS epidemic. Skin involvement can have several presentations. These include superficial lesions of the papillary and upper reticular dermis, which present as reddish or flesh-colored rubbery-to-firm papules, and nodules that resemble pyogenic granulomas and can ulcerate (Fig. 2). The lesions can be found anywhere on the skin, commonly on the upper trunk and face, and occasionally on the anal, oral or gastrointestinal mucosa, or in visceral organs. Some lesions lie deeper in the subcutaneous tissue, are flesh-colored, and can be fixed or mobile. The lesions of bacillary angiomatosis often bleed profusely when traumatized. Bacillary angiomatosis is usually accompanied by fever, ancmia, and elevated erythrocyte sedimentation rate.

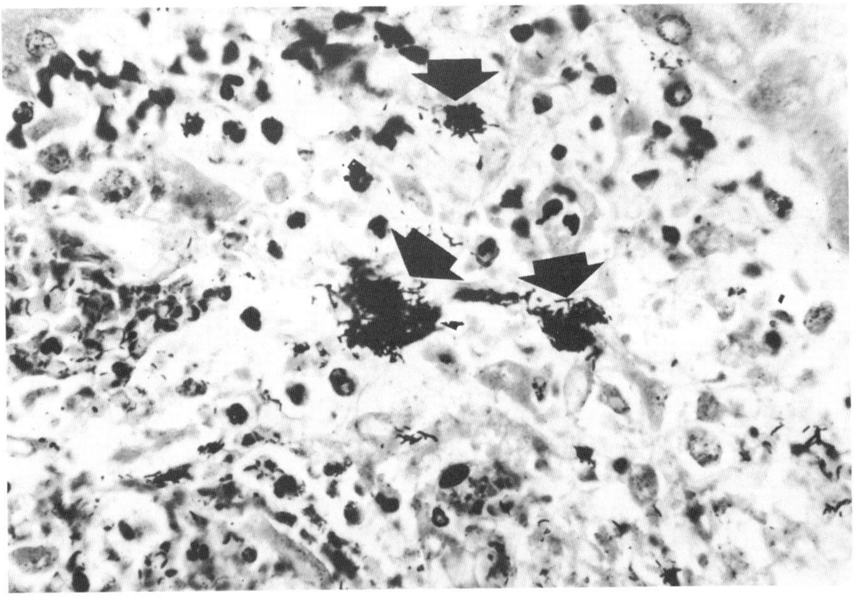

Figure 1

Bacillary angiomatosis. Clusters of bacillary organisms (arrows) are identified on this specimen obtained after Warthin-Starry staining (arrows). (Photograph courtesy of Philip E. Le Boit, M.D.)

Histologic examination of the lesions of bacillary angiomatosis demonstrate circumscribed lobular aggregates of ectatic capillaries lined with protuberant endothelial cells, surrounded by a mucinous stroma with a predominantly neutrophilic inflammatory infiltrate (Fig. 3). They can be mistaken for angiosarcoma due to variable degrees of endothelial cell nuclear atypia and necrosis (22). Although bacillary angiomatosis can also be confused with Kaposi sarcoma (KS) macroscopically, KS is distinct at the microscopic level, characterized by slit-like vessels with spindle-shaped endothelial cells and a lymphocytic inflammatory infiltrate (23,24).

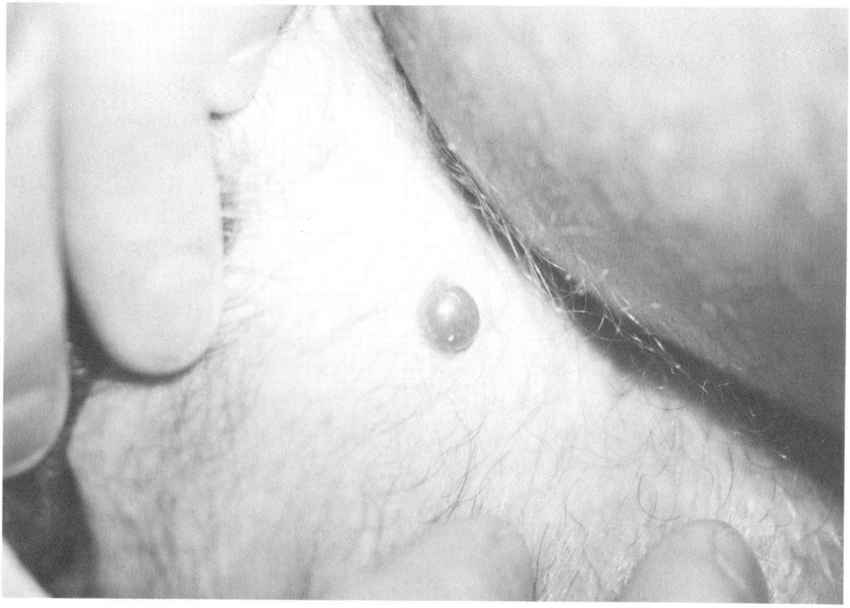

Figure 2

Cutaneous bacillary angiomatosis. Cutaneous lesion of bacillary angiomatosis in a patient with human immunodeficiency virus infection. The rubbery nodule is similar to a pyogenic granuloma. (Photograph courtesy of Philip E. Le Boit, M.D.)

Parenchymal bacillary peliosis manifests as hepatitis and splenitis, which may occur with or without cutaneous lesions (25-28). These visceral lesions are characterized by multiple dilated, blood-filled spaces (peliosis) separated by normal parenchyma and fibromyxoid stroma containing a mixture of neutrophils and mononuclear cells, dilated capillaries, and rod-shaped bacteria in the absence of both vascular proliferation and granuloma formation (7). This appearance is suggestive for the disease, but not specific (29). On CT, one may see numerous hypodense nodules in the liver or spleen. Often there is associated lymphadenopathy (25).

Treatment

The natural history of untreated infection with bacillary angiomatosis is not known. Patients with suspected bacillary angiomatosis or parenchymal peliosis are treated with erythromycin or tetracycline for four to six weeks with good response (26,30,31). Antimicrobial therapy of bacteremic R. henselae infection in both immunocompetent and immunocompromised patients has been frequently associated with relapse, particularly when tetracycline was used. These patients are often given a longer course of treatment. Radiation, intralesional

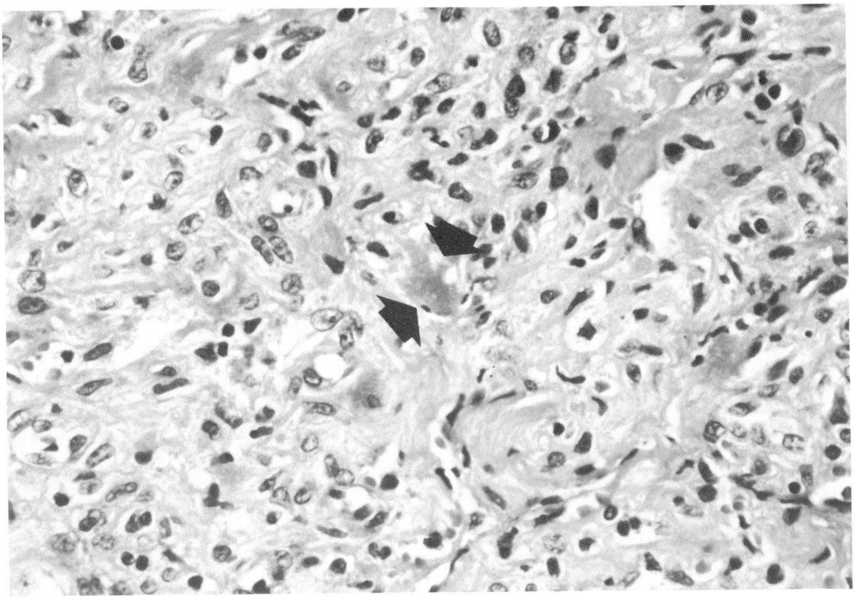

Figure 3

Cutaneous bacillary angiomatosis. A hematoxylin and eosin stain of a biopsy specimen from a skin lesion of bacillary angiomatosis demonstrates a colony of bacteria in the center of the field (arrows). There is a proliferation of capillaries, and an infiltrate of neutrophils and leukocytoclastic debris (hematoxylin and eosin). (Photograph courtesy of Philip E. Le Boit, M.D.)

vinblastine, penicillin, dicloxacillin, cephradine, and nafcillin have no effect on the lesions of bacillary angiomatosis (1).

Skeletal Lesions of Bacillary Angiomatosis

An unusual form of osteomyelitis, caused by bacillary angiomatosis has been seen in HIV-positive patients (2,15,21,30,32,33). The lesions are osteolytic and are frequently associated with an overlying soft tissue mass and periostitis (Figs. 4-9). They demonstrate increased uptake on Technetium-99m methylene diphosphonate scans and are occasionally identified with bone scintigraphy without symptoms or positive findings on radiographs. For this reason, bone scintigraphy is recommended for patients with skin lesions of bacillary angiomatosis. We originally described six of 17 patients (35%) with cutaneous bacillary angiomatosis who had associated osseous lesions (21). Since then, we have encountered two more patients with bacillary angiomatosis in the tibia and skull that healed with antibiotic treatment. The significance of biopsying the lesion and identifying the organism with Warthin-Starry staining is that the patient can be treated with antibiotics, such as erythromycin, with healing and resolution of the lesions.

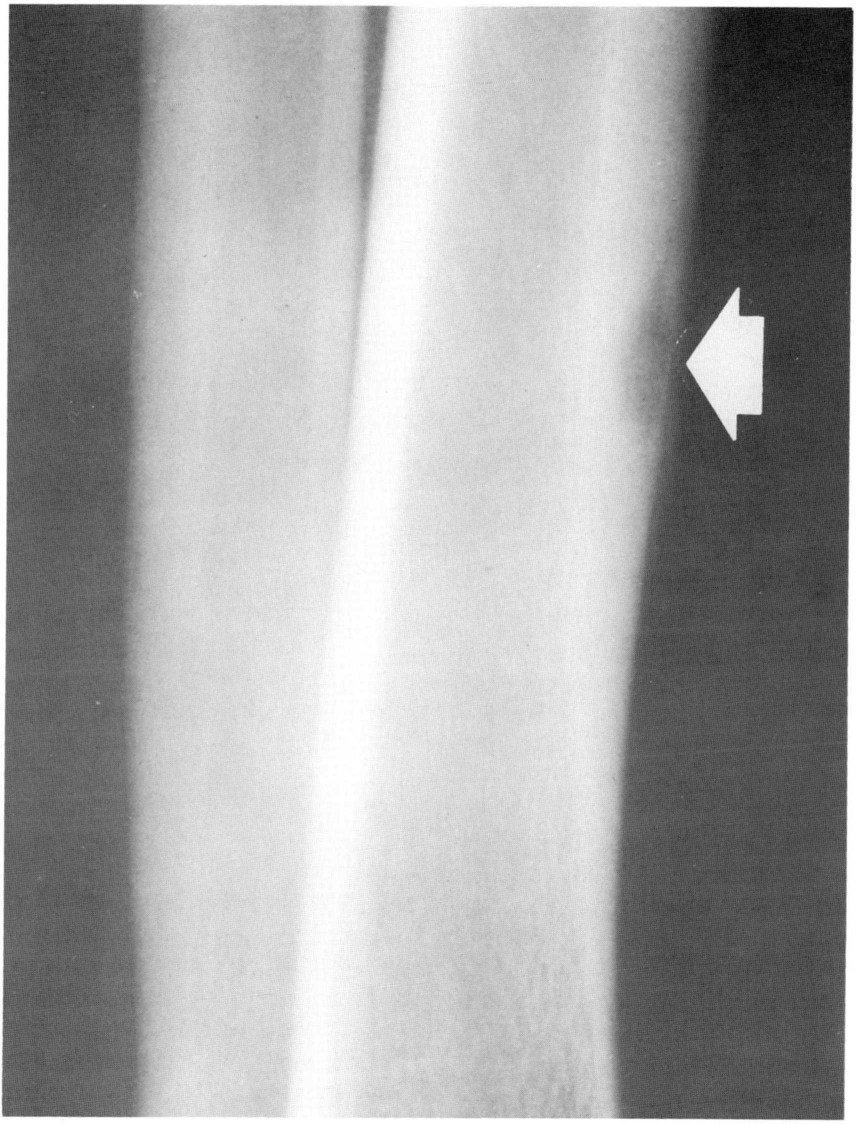

Figure 4

Cutaneous & tibal bacillary angiomatosis. 51-year-old man with pain in the tibia and skin lesions positive for bacillary angiomatosis. Conventional radiographs demonstrated a 1 cm lytic lesion in the distal tibial diaphysis associated with overlying single-layered periostitis (arrow). There was improvement in symptoms and the radiographic appearance of the lesion following antibiotic therapy with erythromycin. (From Baron AL: Radiology 1990;177:77-81, with permission.)

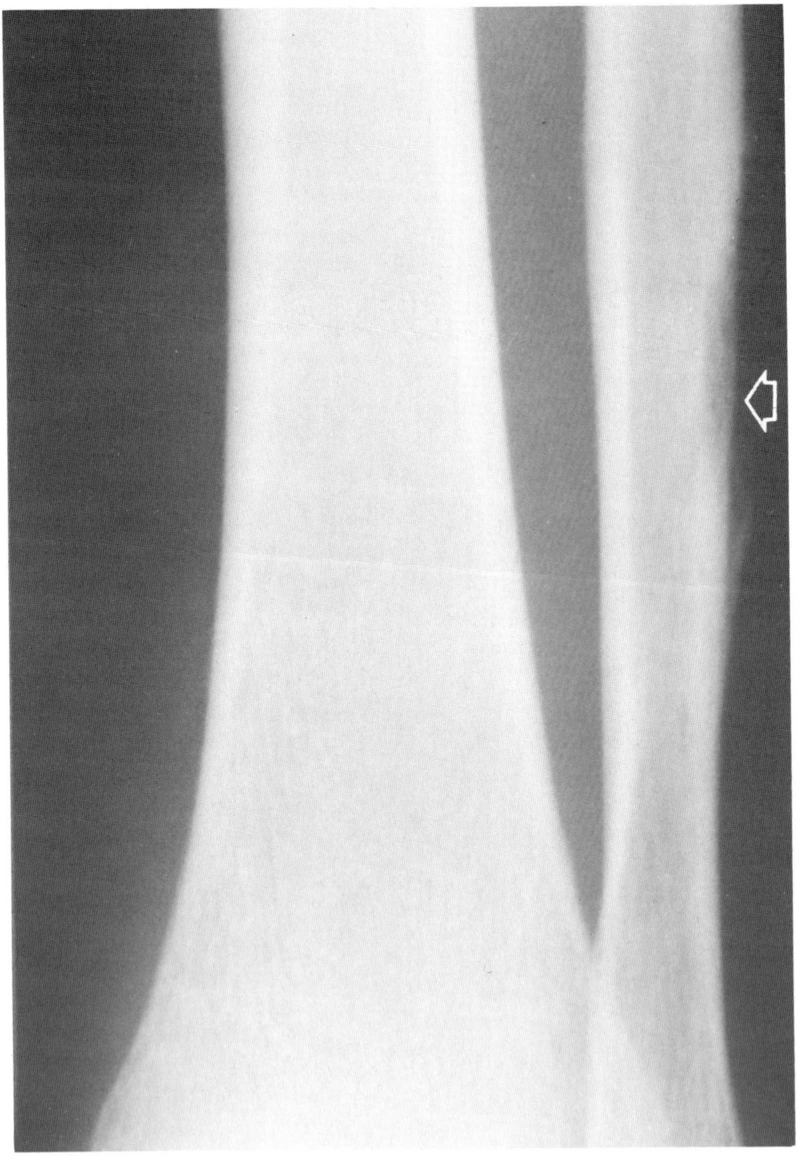

Figure 5

Cutaneous & fibular bacillary angiomatosis. Bacillary angiomatosis in the fibula. An AP radiograph of the fibula reveals an oval, well-circumscribed lytic lesion in the lateral fibular cortex (arrow). Bacillary angiomatosis was also present in the skin overlying the lesion. (From Steinbach LS: Radiology 1993;186:833-838, with permission.)

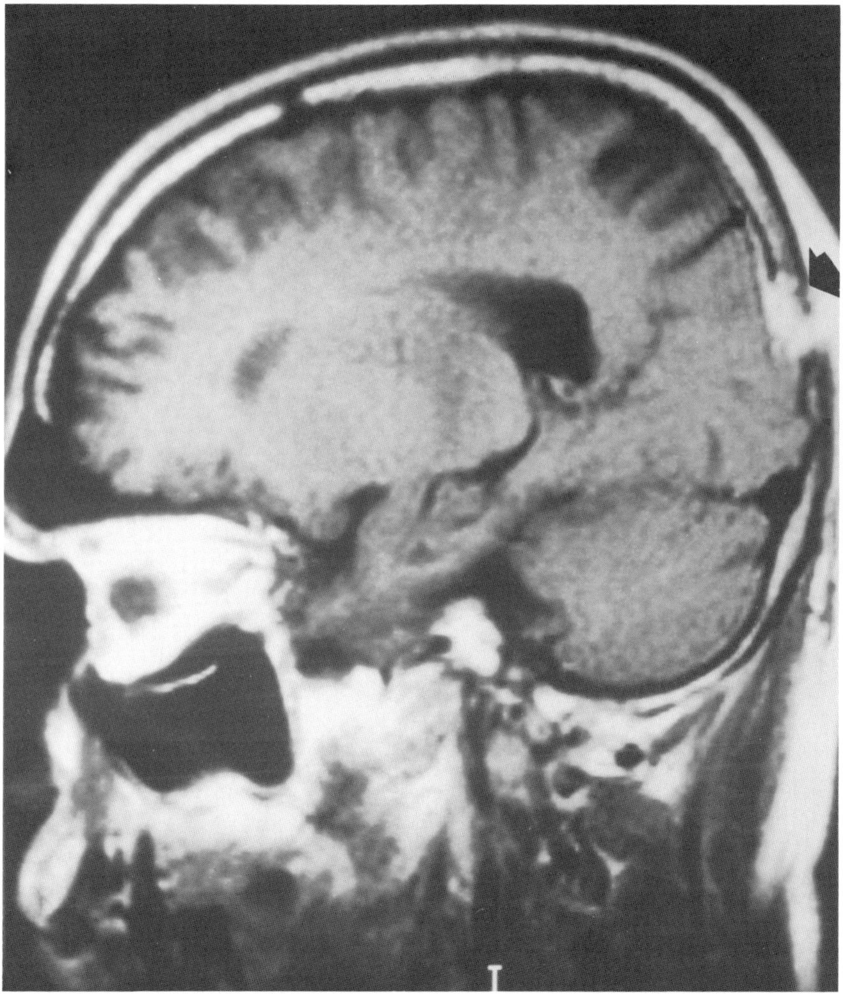

Figure 6-A

Cutaneous & cranial bacillary angiomatosis. Bacillary angiomatosis in the skull. This patient had a lesion which extended from the skin through the occipital bone and into the brain. The lesion enhances on a sagittal T1-weighted MR image (TR=350; TE=25) obtained following gadolinium administration (arrow).

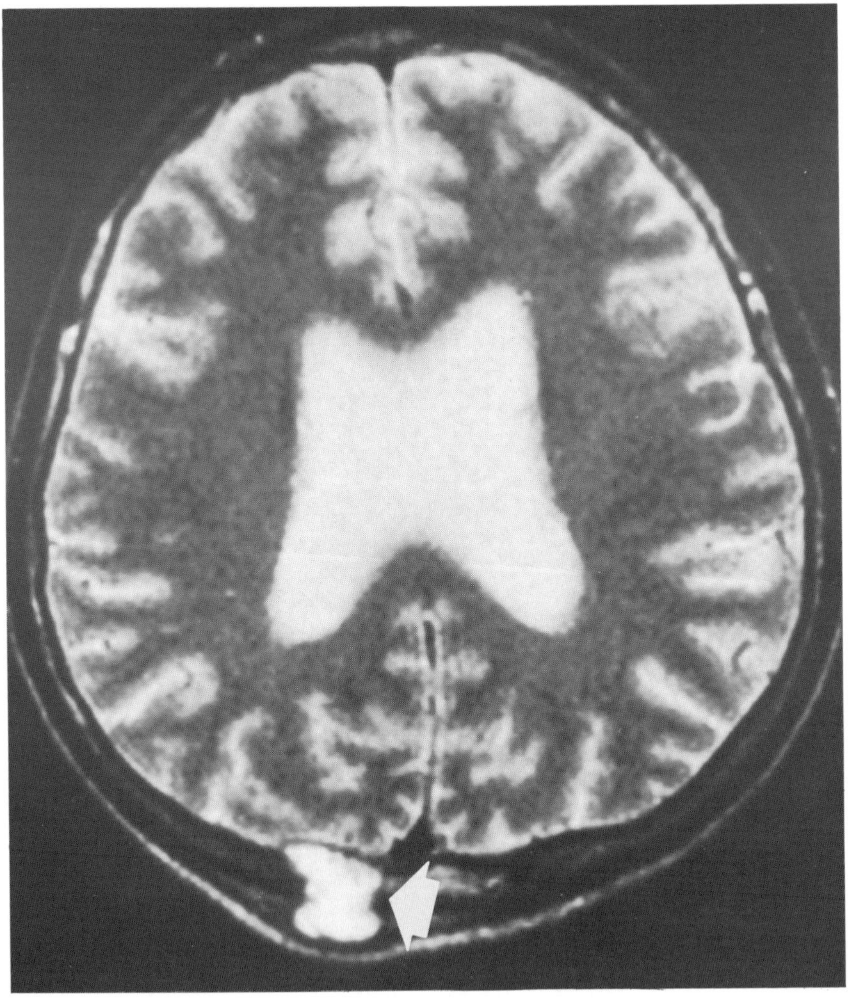

Figure 6-B

The lesion is high signal intensity on an axial T2-weighted (TR=2000; TE=80) MR image (arrow).

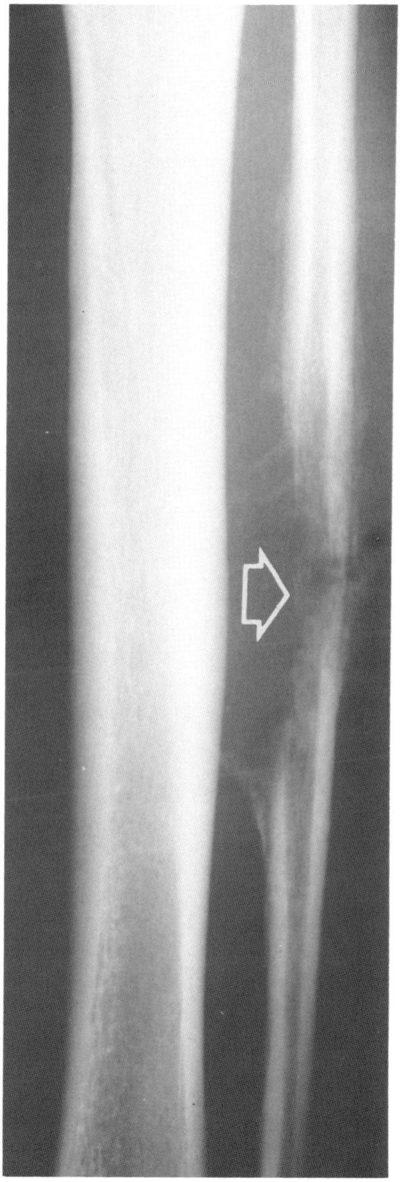

Figure 7-A

Soft tissue & fibular bacillary angiomatosis. Bacillary angiomatosis causes an aggressive destructive lesion which invades the fibular diaphysis on this AP radiograph (arrow).

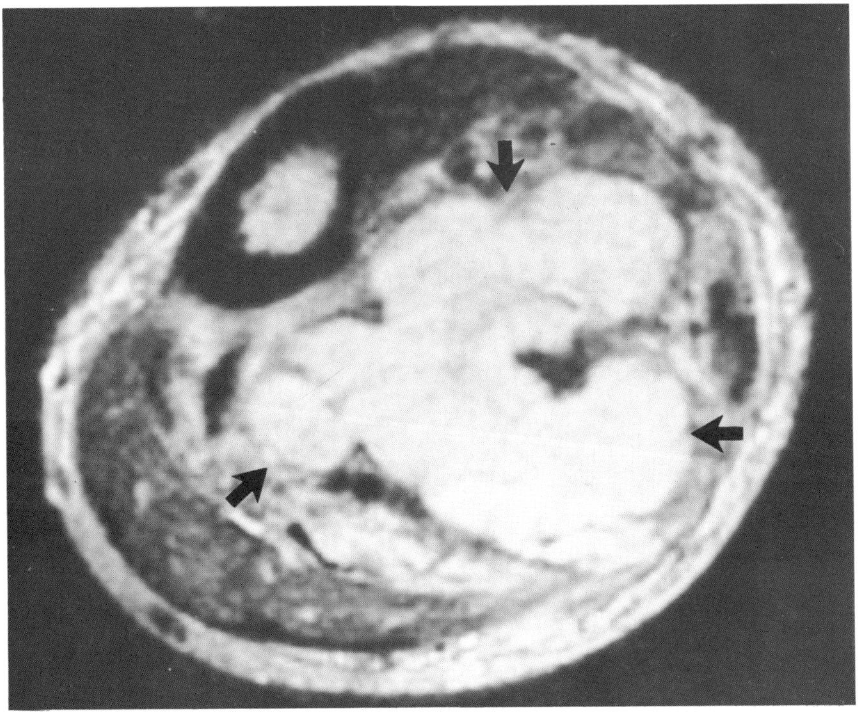

Figure 7-B

A corresponding T2-weighted axial MR image (TR=2000; TE=80) also demonstrates a large high-signal intensity soft-tissue mass that surrounds the fibula and extends into the anterior and posterior compartments of the leg (arrows).

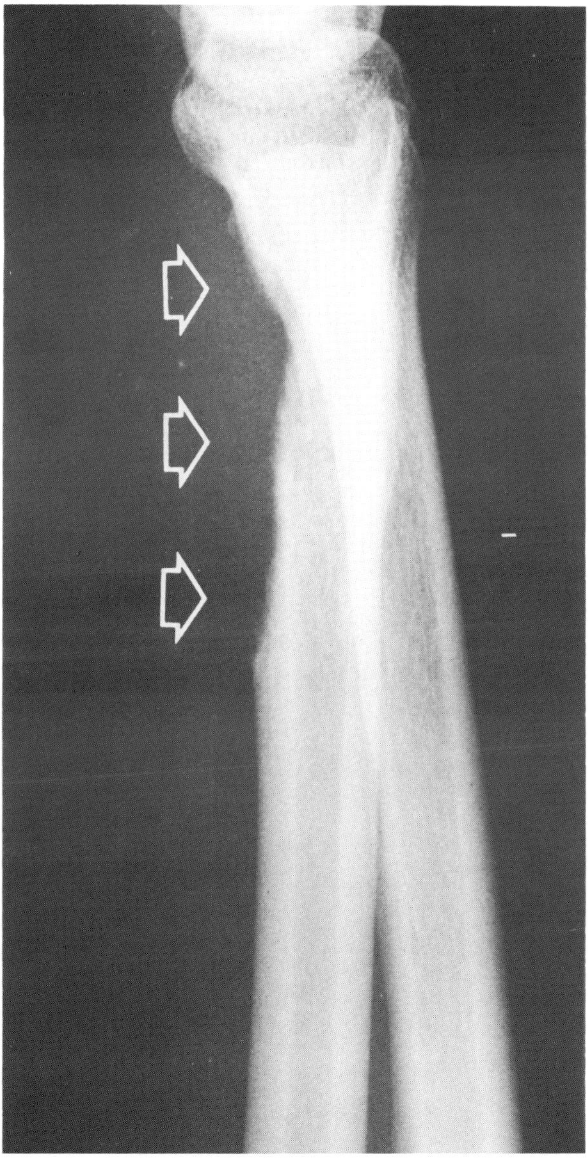

Figure 8-A

Bacillary angiomatosis of soft tissue & radius. This 44-year-old male had bacillary angiomatosis which presented as a mass over the right wrist, causing erosion of the volar aspect of the distal radius (arrows).

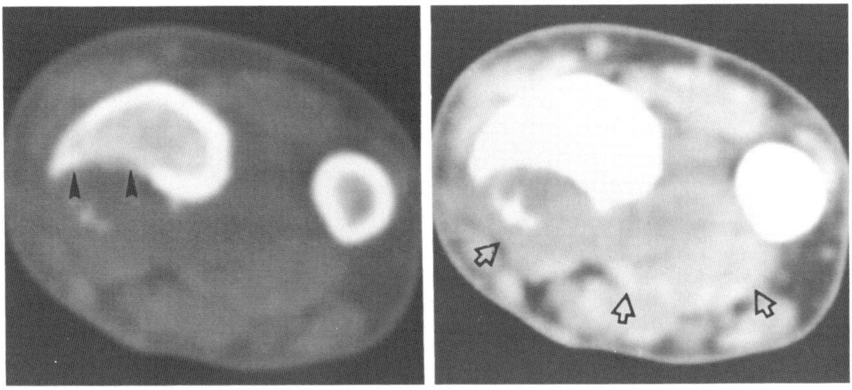

Figure 8-B

Axial CT scan through the area with bone and soft tissue windows demonstrates the cortical destruction (arrowheads) as well as the overlying soft tissue mass (arrows). (From Baron AL: *Radiology* 1990;177:77-81, with permission).

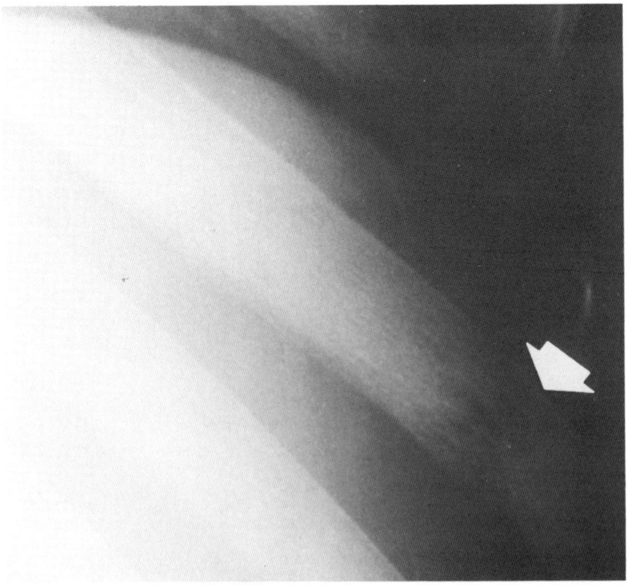

Figure 9-A

Bacillary angiomatosis of thoracic cage. This 30-year-old male had bacillary angiomatosis which presented as a permeative lesion in the left 7th rib (arrow).

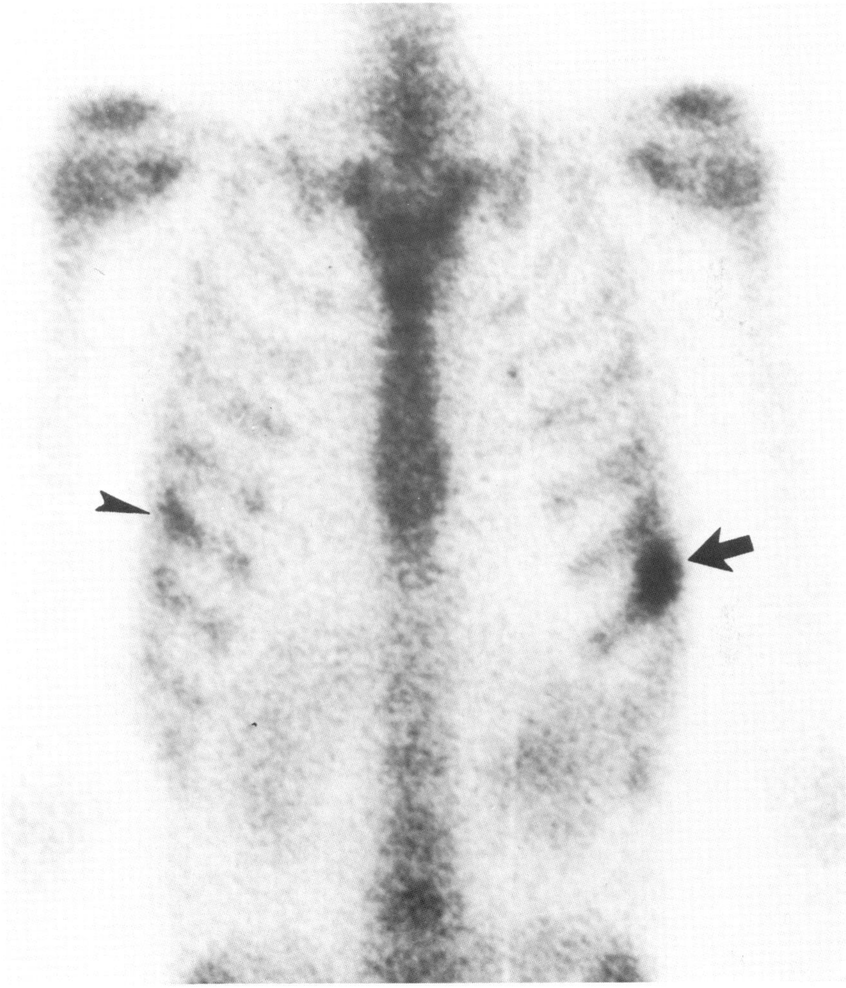

Figure 9-B
The lesion demonstrated high uptake on a Tc-99m-MDP bone scan (arrow). There was also increased uptake in the right 6th rib, consistent with an occult osseous lesion (arrowhead).

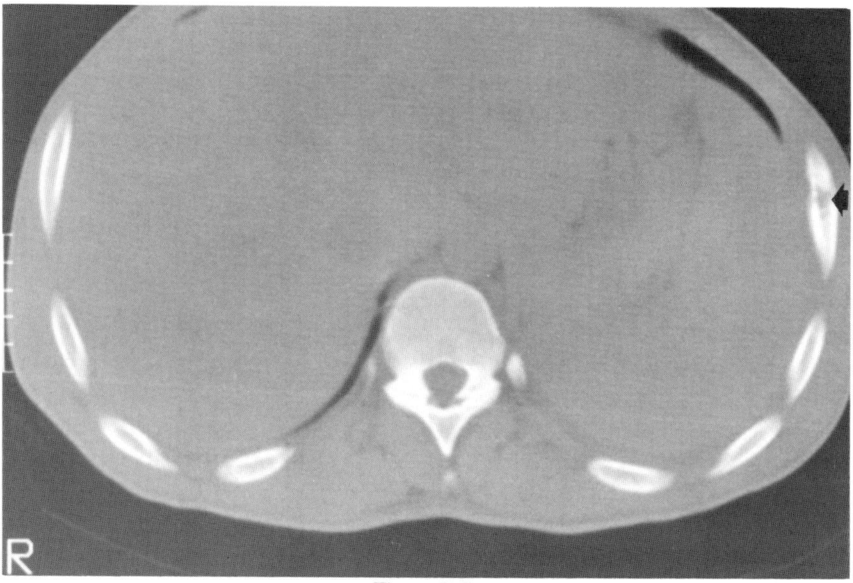

Figure 9-C
There is a lytic defect of the rib on this CT scan obtained with bone windows (arrow).

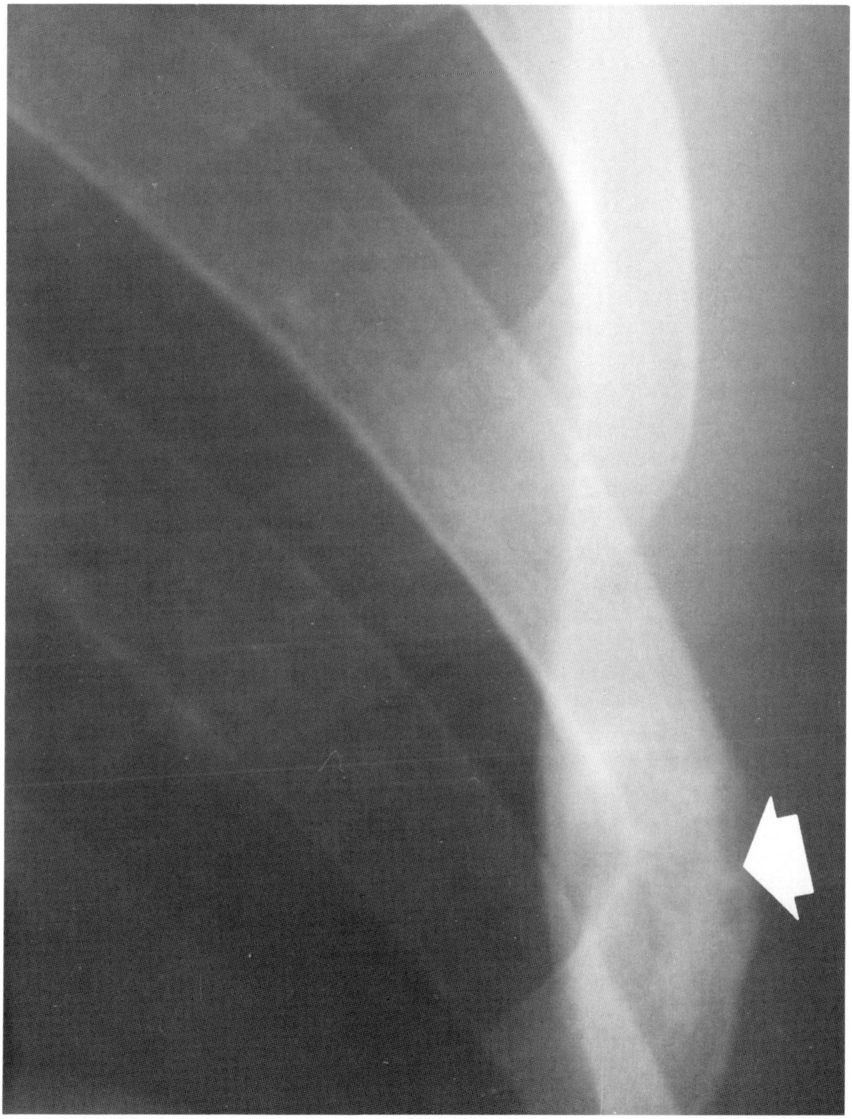

Figure 9-D
The lesion healed after two months of antibiotic therapy (arrow). (From Baron AL: *Radiology* 1990;177:77-81, with permission).

REFERENCES

1. Koehler JE, Quinn FD, Berger TG, LeBoit PE, Tappero JW. Isolation of Rochalimaea species from cutaneous and osseous lesions of bacillary angiomatosis. *NEJM* 1992; 327:1625-1631.
2. LeBoit PE, Berger TG, Egbert BM, Yen TS, Stoler MH, Bonfiglio TA, et al. Epithelioid haemangioma-like vascular proliferation in AIDS: manifestation of cat-scratch disease bacillus infection? *Lancet* 1988;1:960-963.
3. Regnery RL, Anderson BE, Clarridge JE III, Rodriguez-Barradas MC, Jones DC, Carr JH. Characterization of a novel Rochalimaea species, R. henselae, sp. nov., isolated from blood of a febrile, human immunodeficiency virus-positive patient. *I Clin Microbiol* 1992;30:265-274.
4. Welch DF, Pickett DA, Slater LN, Steigerwalt AG, Brenner DJ. Rochalimaea henselae, sp. nov., a cause of septicemia, bacillary angiomatosis, and parenchymal bacillary peliosis. *J Clin Microbiol* 1992;30:275-280.
5. Dolan MJ, Wong MT, Regnery RL, Jorgensen JH, Garcia M, Peters J, Drehner D. Syndrome of Rochalimaea henselae adenitis suggesting cat-scratch disease. *Ann Int Med* 1993;118:331-336.
6. Cockerell CJ, Bergstresser PR, Myrie-Williams C, Tierno PM. Bacillary epithelioid angiomatosis occurring in an immunocompetent individual. *Arch Dermatol* 1990; 126:787-790.
7. Tappero JW, Koehler JE, Berger TG, et al. Bacillary angiomatosis and bacillary splenitis in immunocompetent adults. *Ann Int Med* 1993;118:363-365.
8. Slater LN, Welch DR, Hensel D, Coody DW. A newly recognized fastidious gram-negative pathogen as a cause of fever and bacteremia. *NEJM* 1990;323:1587-1593.
9. Lucey D, Dolan MJ, Moss CW, Garcia M, Hollis DG, Wegner S, et al. Relapsing illness due to Rochalimaea henselae in immunocompetent hosts: implication for therapy and new epidemiological associations. *Clin Infect Dis* 1992;14:383-388.
10. Howe C. Carrion's disease: immunologic studies. *Arch Int Med* 1943;72:147-167.
11. Pchenichkov AV. Results of many years' combined study of trench fever. *J Microbiol Epidemiol Immunobiol* 1957;28:1392-1397.
12. Varela G, Vinson JW, Molina-Pasquel C. Trench fever. II. Propagation of Rickettsia quintana on cell-free medium from the blood of two patients. *Am J Trop Med Hyg* 1969;18:708-712.
13. Logan JS. Trench fever in Belfast, and the nature of the "relapsing fevers" in the United Kingdom in the nineteenth century. *Ulster Med J* 1989;53:83-88.

14. Swift HF. Trench fever. *Arch Int Med* 1920;26:76-98.
15. Relman DA, Loutit JS, Schmidt TM, Falkow S, Tompkins LS. The agent of bacillary angiomatosis. An approach to the identification of uncultured pathogens. *NEJM* 1990;323:1573-1580.
16. Wear DJ, Margileth AM, Hadfield TL, Fischer GW, Schlagel CJ, King FM. Cat-scratch disease: a bacterial infection. *Science* 1983;221:1403-1405.
17. Regnery RL, Olson JG, Perkins BA, Bibb W. Serological response to "Rochalimaea henselae" antigen in suspected cat-scratch disease. *Lancet* 1992;339:1443-1445.
18. Regnery R, Martin M, Olson J. Naturally-occurring "Rochalimaea henselae" infection in domestic cat (Letter). *Lancet* 1992;340:557-558.
19. Brenner DJ, Hollis DG, Moss CW, English CK, Hall GS, Vincent J, et al. Proposal of Afipia gen. nov., with Afipia felis sp. nov. (formerly the Cat Scratch Disease Bacillus), Afipia clevelandensis so. nov. (formerly the Cleveland Clinic Foundation strain), Afipia broomeae sp. nov., and three unnamed genospecies. *J Clin Microbiol* 1991;29:2450-2460.
20. Schlossberg D, Morad Y, Krouse TB, Wear DJ, English CK. Culture-proved disseminated cat-scratch disease in acquired immunodeficiency syndrome. *Arch Int Med* 1989;140:1437-1439.
21. Baron AL, Steinbach LS, LeBoit PE, Mills CM, Gee JH, Berger TG. Osteolytic lesions and bacillary angiomatosis in HIV infection: radiologic differentiation from AIDS-related Kaposi sarcoma. *Radiology* 1990;177:77-81.
22. Tompkins DC, Steigbigel RT. Rochalimaea's role in cat-scratch disease and bacillary angiomatosis. *Ann Int Med* 1993;109:388-390.
23. Cockerell CJ, LeBoit PE. Bacillary angiomatosis: a newly characterized, pseudoneoplastic, infectious, cutaneous vascular disorder. *J Am Acad Dermatol* 1990; 22:501-512.
24. Walford N, Van Der Wouw PA, Ten Velden JJAM, Hulsebosch HJ. Epithelioid angiomatosis in the acquired immunodeficiency syndrome: morphology and differential diagnosis. *Histopathology* 1990;16:83-88.
25. Goodman P, Balachandran S. Bacillary angiomatosis in a patient with HIV infection (Letter). *AJR* 1993;160:207.
26. Perkocha LA, Geaghan SM, Yen TS, Nishimura SL, Chan SP, Garcia-Kennedy R, et al. Clinical and pathological features of bacillary peliosis hepatis in association with human immunodeficiency virus infection. *NEJM* 1990;323:1581-1586.
27. Radin DR, Kanel GC. Peliosis hepatis in a patient with human immunodeficiency virus infection. *AJR* 1991;156:91-92.
28. Radin DR. Spontaneous resolution of peliosis of the liver and spleen in a patient with HIV infection (Letter). *AJR* 1992;158:1409.
29. Carithers HA. Cat-scratch disease: an overview based on a study of 1200 patients. *Am J Dis Child* 1985;139:1124-1133.

30. Koehler JE, LeBoit PE, Egbert BM, Berger TG. Cutaneous vascular lesions and disseminated cat-scratch disease in patients with the acquired immunodeficiency syndrome (AIDS) and AIDS-related complex. *Ann Int Med* 1988;109:449-455.
31. Rudikoff D, Phelps RG, Gordon RE, Bottone EJ. Acquired immunodeficiency syndrome-related bacillary vascular proliferation (epithelioid angiomatosis): rapid response to erythromycin therapy (Letter). *Arch Dermatol* 1989;125:706-707.
32. LeBoit PE, Berger T, Egbert BM, Beckstead JH, Yen TB, Stoler M. Bacillary angiomatosis: the histopathology and differential diagnosis of a pseudoneoplastic infection in patients with HIV infection. *Am J Surg Pathol* 1989;13:909-920.
33. Herts BR, Rafii M, Spiegel G. Soft tissue and osseous lesions caused by bacillary angiomatosis: unusual manifestations of cat-scratch fever in patients with AIDS. *AJR* 1991;157:1249-1251.

CHAPTER 3:

TUBERCULOSIS AND OTHER ATYPICAL MYCOBACTERIAL INFECTIONS IN AIDS PATIENTS

Jamshid Tehranzadeh, M.D.
Carol H. Wong, M.D.

EPIDEMIOLOGY

Since 1985, the number of cases of tuberculosis has been on the rise in the United States. Several lines of epidemiological evidence support this resurgence of tuberculosis related to the HIV (Human Immunodeficiency Virus) epidemic. In the general population, apparent tuberculosis develops in approximately 10% of infected individuals, either soon after primary infection or years later (reactivation TB). Patients with HIV infection are at a much higher risk for primary or reactivation tuberculosis. Among HIV-infected individuals with positive tuberculin skin tests, the risk of active tuberculosis is estimated to be 8% per year. The incidence of tuberculosis in patients with AIDS is almost 500 times that in the general population (1,2).

GENERAL CLINICAL FEATURES

Tuberculosis is often the first indication of immunodeficiency in patients with HIV infection and usually precedes the diagnosis of AIDS. Clinical presentation reflects the degree of cellular immunity compromise. Recently, highly resistant strains of mycobacterium have been reported in the AIDS population. Tuberculosis in the early stage of HIV infection is usually indistinguishable from that which occurs in the non-HIV-infected person, including preserved cutaneous reactivity to tuberculin and apical pulmonary disease with cavitation. In the later stage of HIV infection, after the diagnosis of AIDS, clinical presentation of tuberculosis is more unusual. There is a loss of cutaneous reactivity to tuberculin. Chest radiographic findings are more common in those with primary tuberculosis. The central nervous system and gastrointestinal tract (including esophageal fistulas and splenic abscesses) can be affected by tuberculosis in patients with AIDS (1-4).

PULMONARY TUBERCULOSIS

Pulmonary involvement occurs in 74% of all patients with HIV infection who have tuberculosis. Early in the course of HIV infection, findings on chest radiographs are those of reactivation tuberculosis with apical cavitary disease similar to that seen in non-HIV-infected individuals with reactivation TB. As the disease progresses, with increasing degree of immunocompromise, radiologic findings appear more typical of primary tuberculosis. These findings consist of mediastinal or hilar adenopathy, noncavitary abnormalities in any lung zone, often with a miliary pattern, and pleural effusions (1-3,5).

GASTROINTESTINAL TUBERCULOSIS

Tuberculosis of the GI tract involves the ileocecal area 90% of the time. Clinical presentation usually includes chronic diarrhea, fever and abdominal pain. Radiologically, the ileocecal valve is thickened and ulcers are frequently found in the mucosa of the ileocecal region. The cecum is usually involved with spiculation, stenosis and retraction. The terminal ileum may become fibrotic, with the ileocecal valve becoming rigid and incontinent (6). Rarely, the duodenum is involved. Fold thickening and widening of the duodenal loop may be observed. Duodenal fistulas may occur.

Involvement of the esophagus has also been reported (7). Barium esophagram and CT demonstrate deep ulceration and transmural communication, including esophagobronchial fistulization and sinus tracts from the esophagus to adjacent necrotic, infected lymph nodes. Esophageal involvement is thought to be secondary to spread from the adjacent infected mediastinal nodes.

Other intraabdominal involvement includes the peritoneum, lymphatic ganglia and solid viscera (liver and spleen). Free or loculated ascitic fluid may be seen. Adenopathy in the peripancreatic area, mesentery, and near the involved intestinal segments is often observed. Lymph nodes demonstrate peripheral enhancement following contrast injection with hypodense centers, which are probably due to necrotic caseation.

CENTRAL NERVOUS SYSTEM TUBERCULOSIS

Tuberculosis causes meningitis, chronic tuberculoma, and, rarely, multiple brain abscesses (8). Calcification in chronic or healing tuberculoma is best seen by CT. Both CT and MR demonstrate infarction caused by tuberculous meningitis, which often involves the territories supplied by the lenticulostriate arteries. Meningitis is best seen on gadopentatate dimeglumine-enhanced Tl-weighted MR images. There is also abnormal enhancement in the basal cisterns.

MYCOBACTERIUM AVIUM COMPLEX

This is a group of atypical mycobacteria which are potentially pathogenic and commonly found in the environment. Disseminated disease is the most common form seen in AIDS patients. The diagnosis of disseminated M. avium complex is usually made late in the course of HIV infection, often in conjunction with or after the occurrence of at least one other opportunistic infection (2). Clinical symptoms that have been attributed to M. avium complex are non-specific and may include intermittent fever, weight loss, cachexia, and gastro-intestinal symptoms ranging from vague abdominal pain to chronic diarrhea and significant malabsorption. M. avium complex has been isolated from bone marrow, lymph nodes, lung, gastrointestinal tract, liver, spleen, urine, and blood.

SKELETAL TUBERCULOSIS

Tuberculous involvement of the musculoskeletal system was infrequent even in the days when pulmonary TB was common, occurring in only approximately 3% to 5% of patients, although a much higher frequency, approximately 30%, was seen in patients with extrapulmonary tuberculosis (9,10). It is generally accepted that skeletal tuberculosis occurs mainly by hematogenous spread. Seeding of the skeleton may arise from a primary infection of the lung or, at a later date, from a quiescent primary site or an extraosseous focus. Skeletal lesions result from implantation of the bacilli in the medullary bone. Classically, the vertebral column is most commonly affected. In other bones, metaphyseal involvement is perhaps more common. Hips and knees are the most commonly affected joints. Diagnosis is confirmed by demonstration of tubercle bacilli in smear or culture and may require closed or open biopsy of bone and aspiration of the joint or biopsy of the synovial membrane.

Tuberculous Spondylitis

The thoracic and lumbar spine are most commonly affected, especially the first lumbar vertebra. Involvement of the cervical spine and sacrum are uncommon, although involvement of the sacroiliac joint is not rare. Infection most often begins in the anterior portion of the vertebral body, then spreads to involve the intervertebral disc and neighboring vertebral body. Posterior elements may be initially or predominantly affected in some individuals, but this is much less common.

Radiologically, there is bony destruction involving the vertebral body anteriorly, narrowing of the adjacent intervertebral disc and similar bone destruction of the contiguous vertebral body. The end-plates adjacent to the affected intervertebral disc lose their definition and, eventually, progressive vertebral collapse with anterior wedging leads to the characteristic gibbus formation.

There is frequent ligamentous and soft tissue extension from the vertebrae and discs, usually anterolaterally and, rarely, posteriorly into the peridural space. In the lumbar region, a psoas abscess may form which can extend into the groin and thigh. Paravertebral abscesses may penetrate the esophagus, bronchus, mediastinum, liver, kidney, intestine, bladder, rectum, vagina, and aorta. Psoas abscesses may contain calcification. Clinically, there may be spinal cord compression causing paralysis from abscesses, granulation tissue, bone fragments, arachnoiditis, and ischemia of the cord.

We have encountered a multicentric (disseminated) form of musculoskeletal tuberculosis in a 30-year-old HIV-positive patient (Fig. 1). Ultrasound and CT can provide important information in patients with psoas or paraspinal abscesses. Magnetic resonance imaging (11) enables prediction of the presence of neurologic complication in 93% of patients and diagnosis of the type of infection in 94%. Vertebral intraosseous abscesses, meningeal involvement, subligamentous spread, and paraspinal abscess location are best identified on contrast-enhanced studies. High signal intensities on T1-weighted images of previously affected vertebrae suggest healing and correlated well with symptoms.

Tuberculous Osteomyelitis

Essentially any bone can be affected by tuberculosis (TB). The disease may remain localized to bone or progress to involve adjacent articulation. Radiologically, there are foci of osteolysis with varying amounts of eburnation and periostitis. There is sequestrum formation. The initial appearance is similar to that in other types of osteomyelitis and even an aggressive neoplasm.

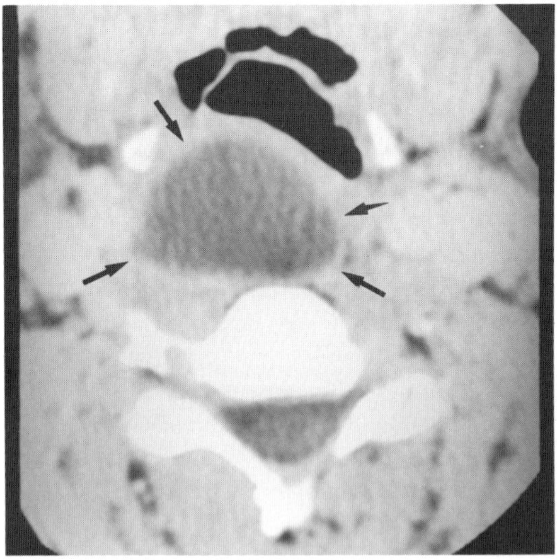

Figure 1-A

Disseminated muscuooskeletal tuberculosis. This is a 30-year-old HIV-positive man with disseminated musculoskeletal tuberculosis. CT scan of the cervical spine at the C4 level (soft tissue window) shows retropharyngeal prevertebral abscess formation (arrows). Note marked displacement of the pharynx at this level. This patient also had lytic changes at C2 and C3 vertebral bodies (not shown here).

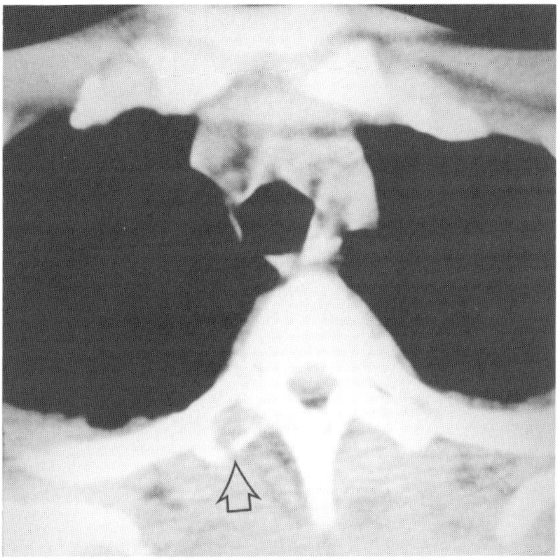

Figure 1-B
Soft tissue window of CT scan of thoracic spine at the T2 level shows lytic lesion in the right transverse process at the costovertebral junction (open arrow).

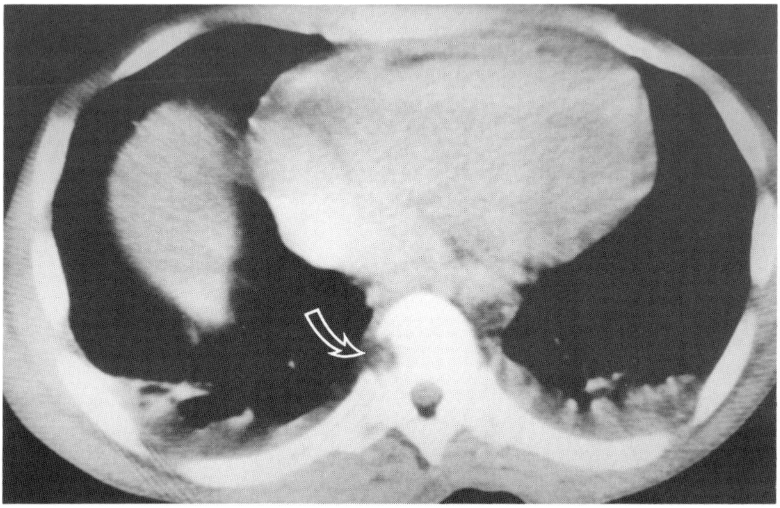

Figure 1-C
Soft tissue window of CT scan of thoracic spine at the cardiac level shows lytic lesion of the vertebral body (open arrow). Note the bilateral pleural effusions and pleural pulmonary reaction due to pulmonary involvement with tuberculosis.

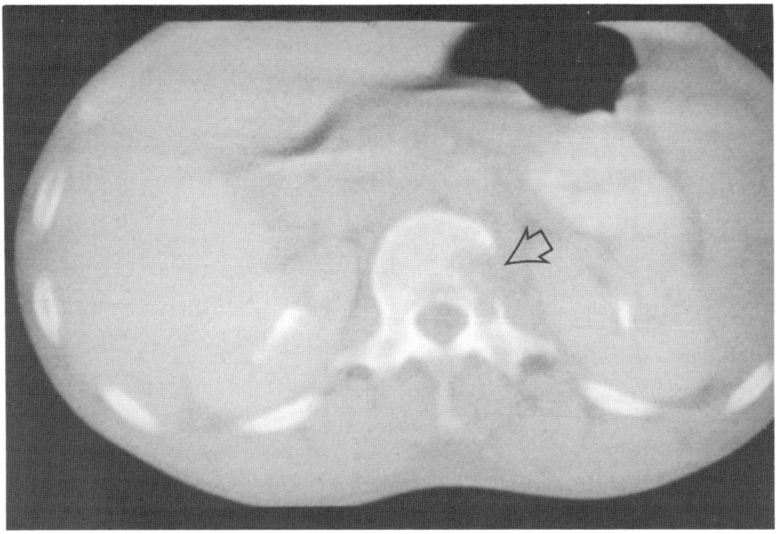

Figure 1-D

Bone window of the CT scan at T12 level shows relatively large lytic lesion involving the body and pedicle of the vertebra on the left side (open arrow).

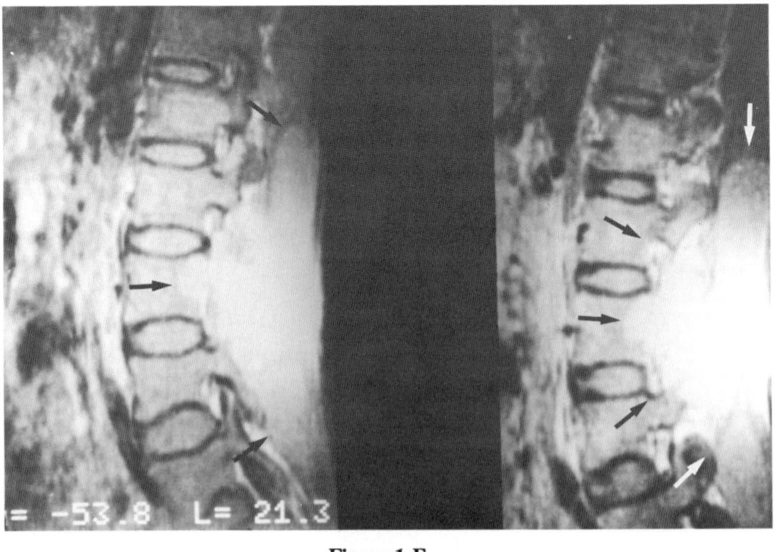

Figure 1-E

Parasagittal T1-weighted images (TR 600, TE 30) shows large posterior epidural abscess involving the posterior elements at L2, L3 and L4 levels and vertebral body at L3 level (arrows). This was contiguous with a psoas abscess. Note generalized decrease in the bone marrow signal intensity throughout the spine.

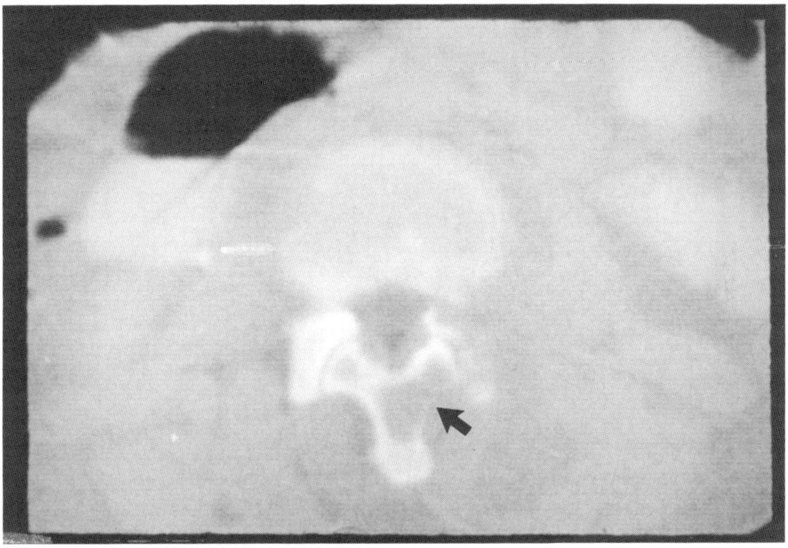

Figure 1-F

CT bone window at the lumbar spine shows lytic lesion of the lamina and the spinous process of L2 vertebra (arrow). Paravertebral and psoas abscess is also noted.

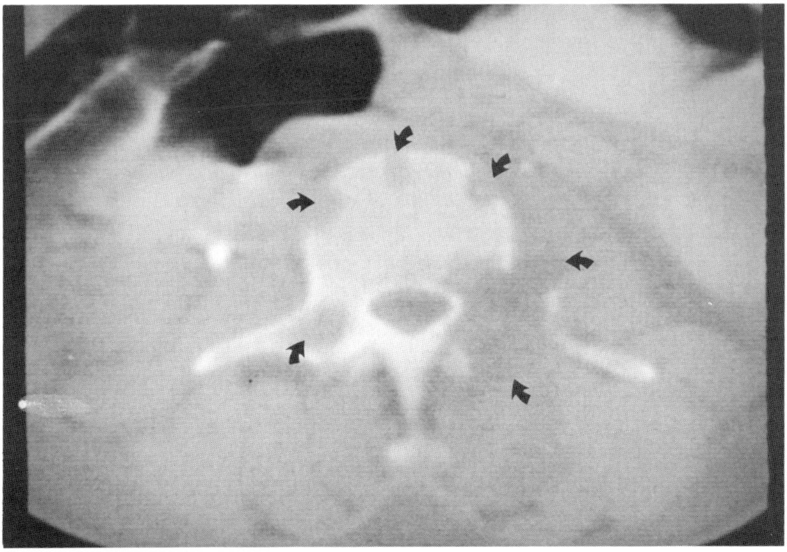

Figure 1-G

CT of lumbar spine (bone window). Multiple lytic lesions of the vertebral body and posterior elements due to paravertebral and psoas abscess are noted (curved arrows).

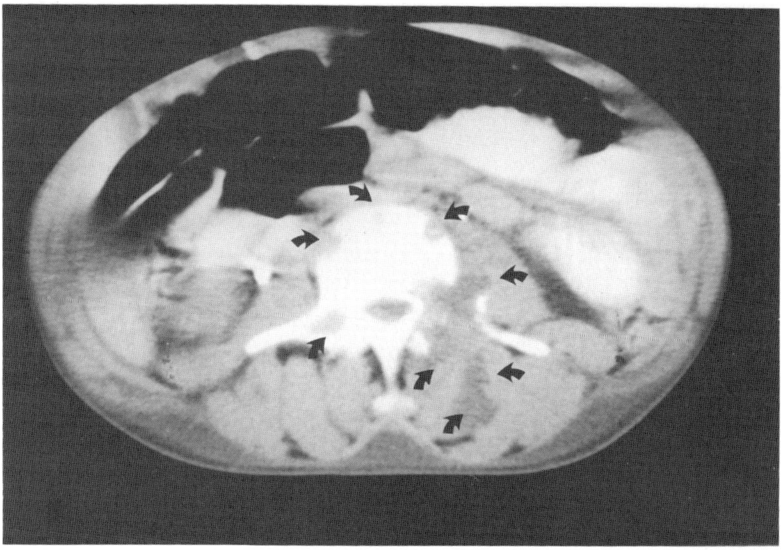

Figure 1-H
CT of lumbar spine (soft tissue window). Multiple lytic lesions of the vertebral body and posterior elements due to paravertebral and psoas abscesses are noted (curved arrows).

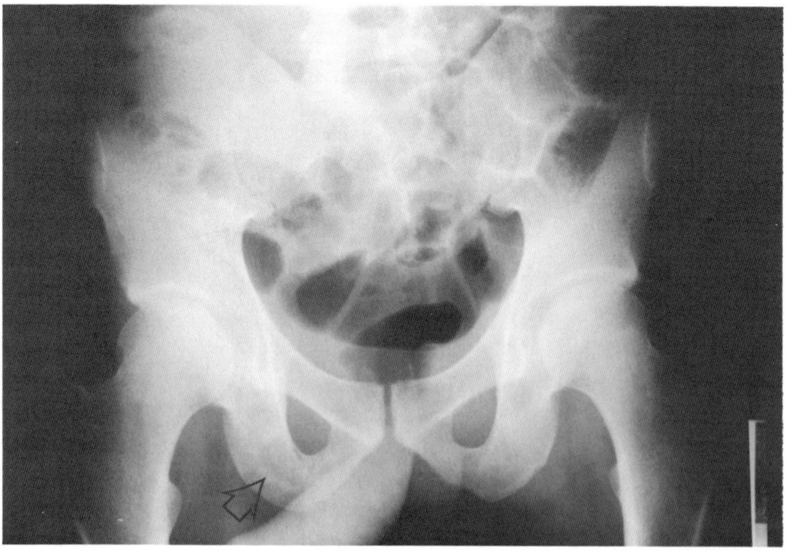

Figure 1-I
Oval well-circumscribed lytic lesion of the right ischial bone (open arrow).

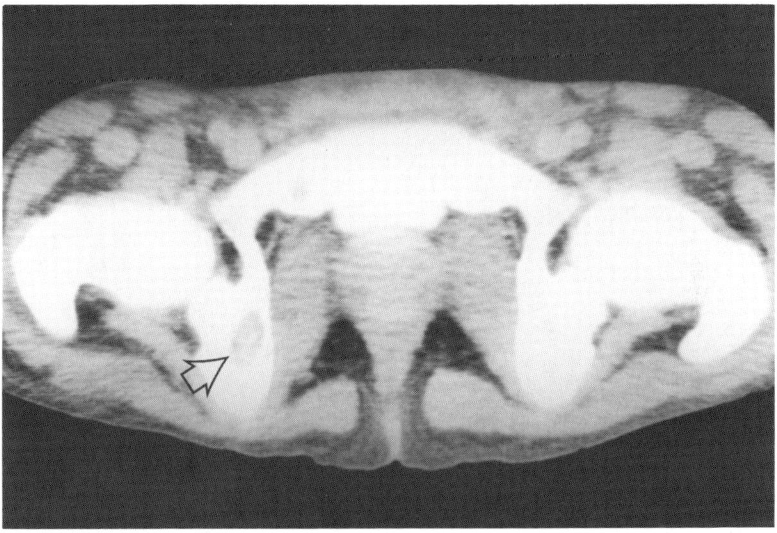

Figure 1-J
CT scan of pelvis (soft tissue window) shows an oval lytic lesion in the right ischial bone (open arrow).

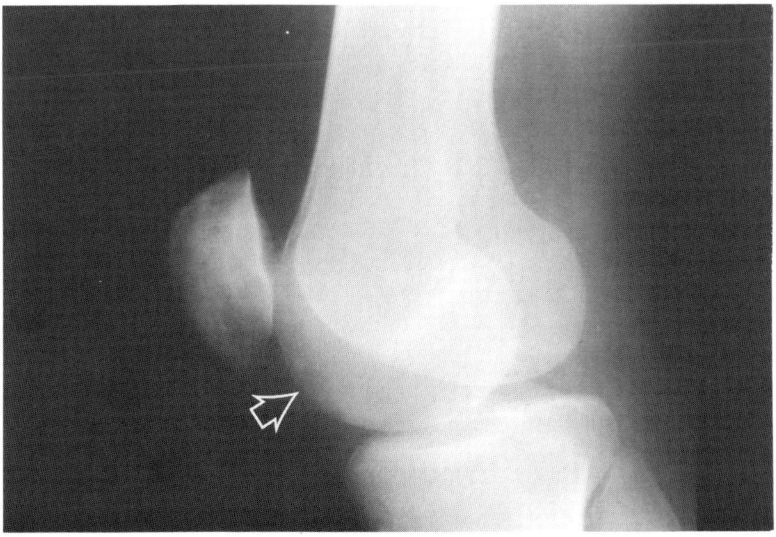

Figure 1-K
Oblique view of the right knee shows joint effusion with cortical erosion of the femoral condyle due to tuberculous arthritis.

Cystic tuberculosis is a special type of TB osteomyelitis. There are disseminated lesions of the axial and extraaxial skeleton. More frequently seen in children than adults, TB usually affects the peripheral skeleton. Lesions may be symmetric in distribution and are of variable size without surrounding sclerosis. We have encountered diffuse ulnar tuberculosis osteomyelitis in a 12-year-old HIV-positive girl (Fig. 2).

Tuberculous dactylitis is seen more frequently in children than in adults. Soft tissue swelling is usually the initial manifestation. There is mild or exuberant periostitis of phalanges, metacarpals or metatarsals. It can have a similar appearance to sickle cell dactylitis and luetic dactylitis. Expansion of bone with cystic quality is termed spina ventosa.

Tuberculous Arthritis

Tuberculous arthritis typically affects large joints and is a monoarticular disease. The majority of joint lesions are secondary to adjacent osteomyelitis. Radiologically, there is a triad of juxtaarticular osteoporosis, peripherally located osseous erosions, and gradual narrowing of the interosseous space (Phemister's triad). The authors previously reported two women with HIV infection, aged 31 and 43 years, who had tuberculous arthritis in the ankle and shoulder, respectively (Figs. 3, 4 & 5) (12).

Atypical Mycobacterial Infection

In atypical mycobacterial infection, lesions tend to be multiple rather than solitary. Metaphyses and diaphyses of long bones are most commonly affected. They are discrete lesions which may contain sclerotic margins. Osteoporosis may not be as striking as that seen in tuberculous infection. There is a tendency toward the development of abscesses and sinus tracts.

Two cases of mycobacterium avium complex (MAC)-induced arthritis in AIDS patients have been reported (13,14). Blumenthal, et al (14) described a 30-year-old man with AIDS who developed MAC septic arthritis and osteomyelitis of both wrists and feet during the terminal stage of his illness. The patient's clinical course was rapidly progressive and destructive, more characteristic of a bacterial septic arthritis. However, Vinetz, et al (13) reported a 38-year-old man who had chronic arthritis of the left wrist and knee secondary to MAC over one year's duration. There was no bony destruction and the patient was clinically responsive to antimycobacterial therapy.

Mycobacterium haemophilum, an unusual pathogen, has been reported to induce skin infection and septic arthritis in AIDS patients (15,16). M. haemophilum infection was previously found in immunocompromised hosts secondary to renal transplant and Hodgkin's lymphoma. M. haemophilum skin lesions begin as painful erythematous nodules and may progress to form abscesses and ulcerate. M. haemophilum can also cause tenosynovitis of the

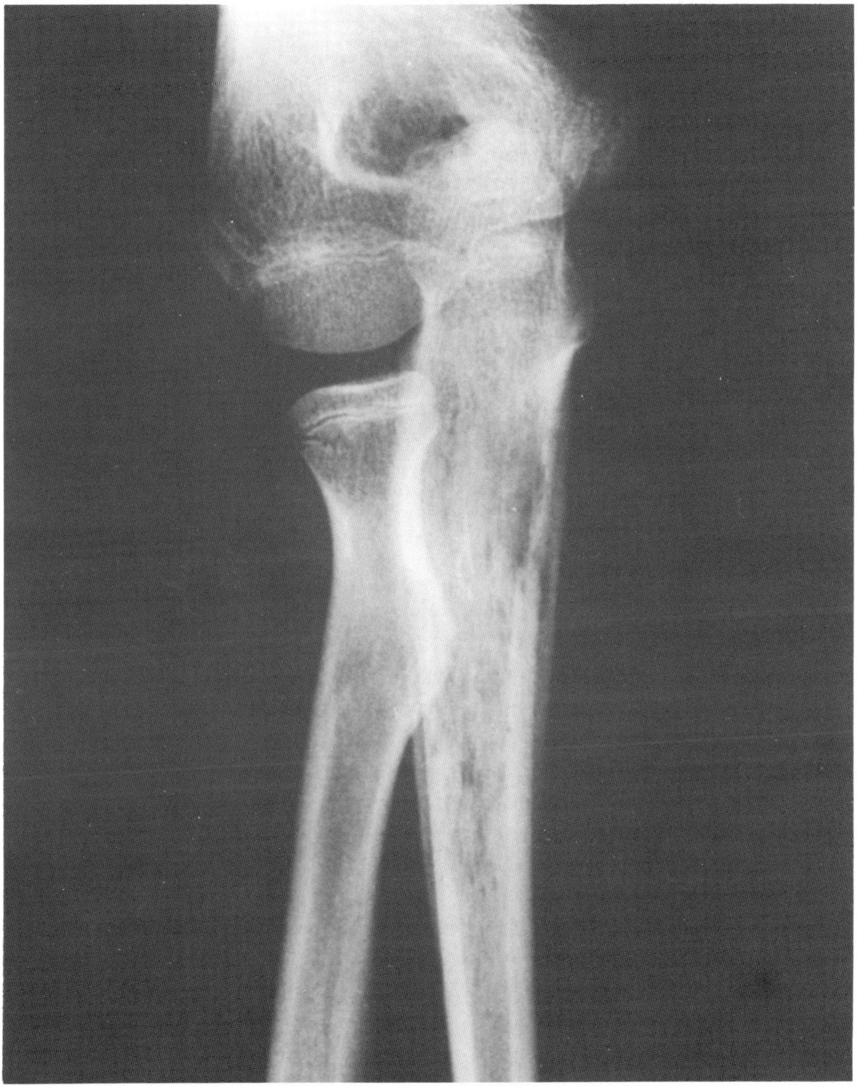

Figure 2-A

Tuberculosis osteomyelitis. 12-year-old girl with AIDS and diffuse tuberculous osteomyelitis of the proximal and distal ulna of the right forearm. AP (A) and lateral (B) views of the right forearm show permeative lytic lesions of the proximal ulna with diffuse periosteal reaction on medial and lateral sides of the proximal ulna.

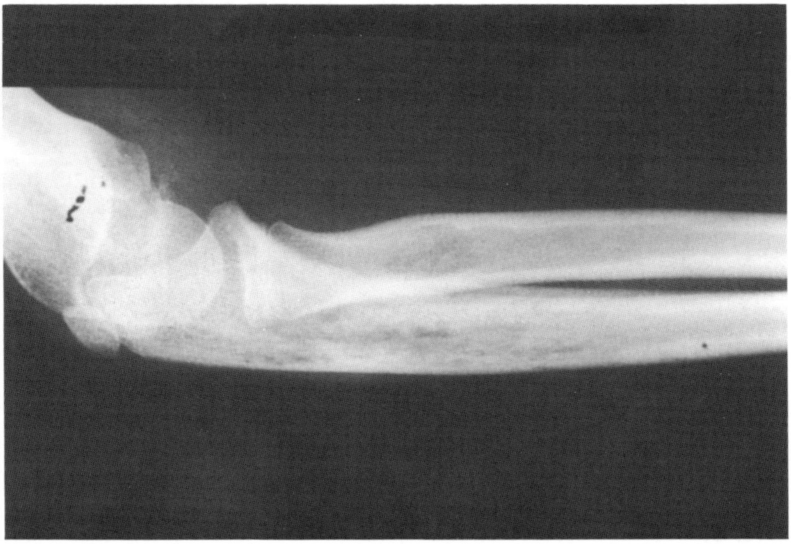

Figure 2-B
AP (A) and lateral (B) views of the right forearm show permeative lytic lesions of the proximal ulna with diffuse periosteal reaction of the proximal ulna.

knee, ankle, wrist, digit, and tendon sheath. Only one out of five reported cases responded to antimycobacterial therapy with clinical improvement.

Pouchot, et al (17) reported a case of tuberculous polymyositis in an HIV-infected individual during an active tuberculous infection. The patient had proximal muscle weakness and elevated creatine kinase (CK). Muscle biopsy revealed granulomata. The patient improved with antimycobacterial therapy. The authors also previously described a patient with tuberculous myositis and sacroiliitis (12).

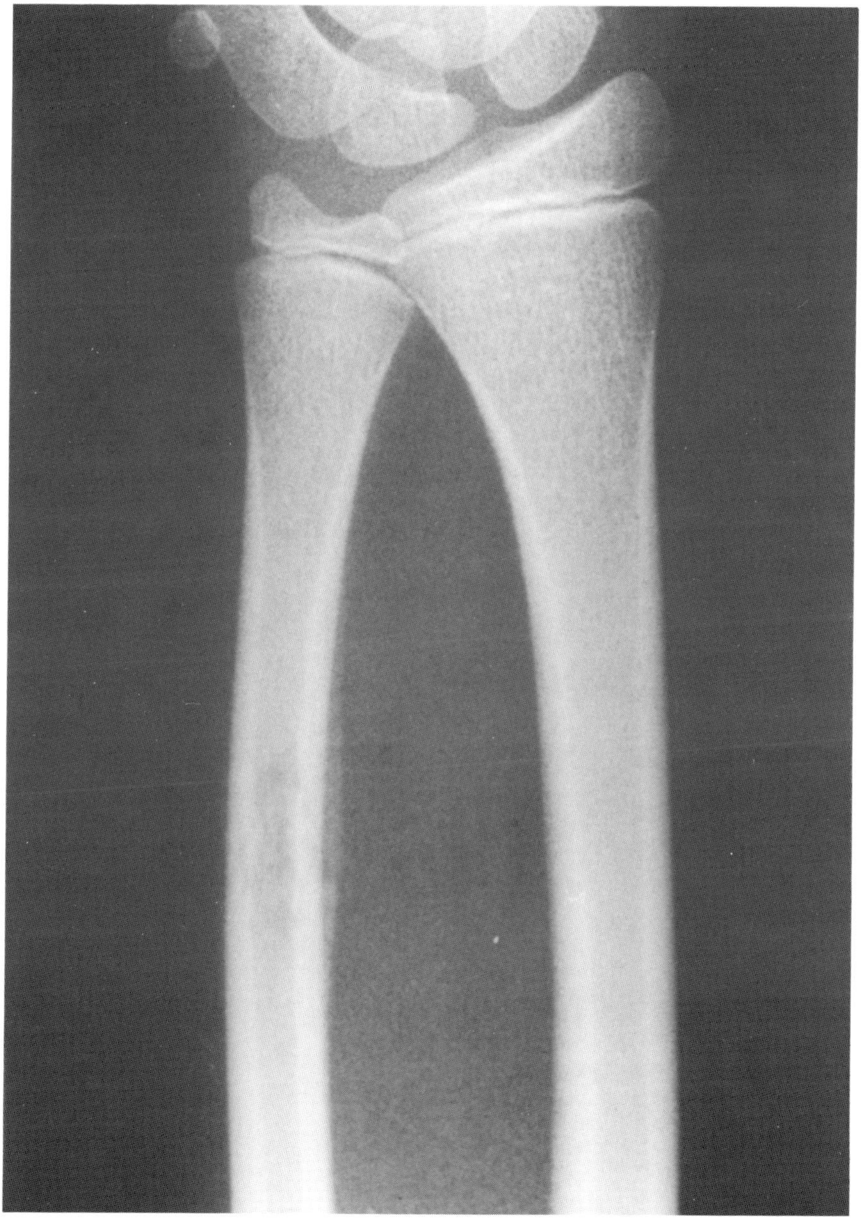

Figure 2-C
AP view of distal forearm shows lytic changes of the distal third of the ulnar shaft with periosteal reaction.

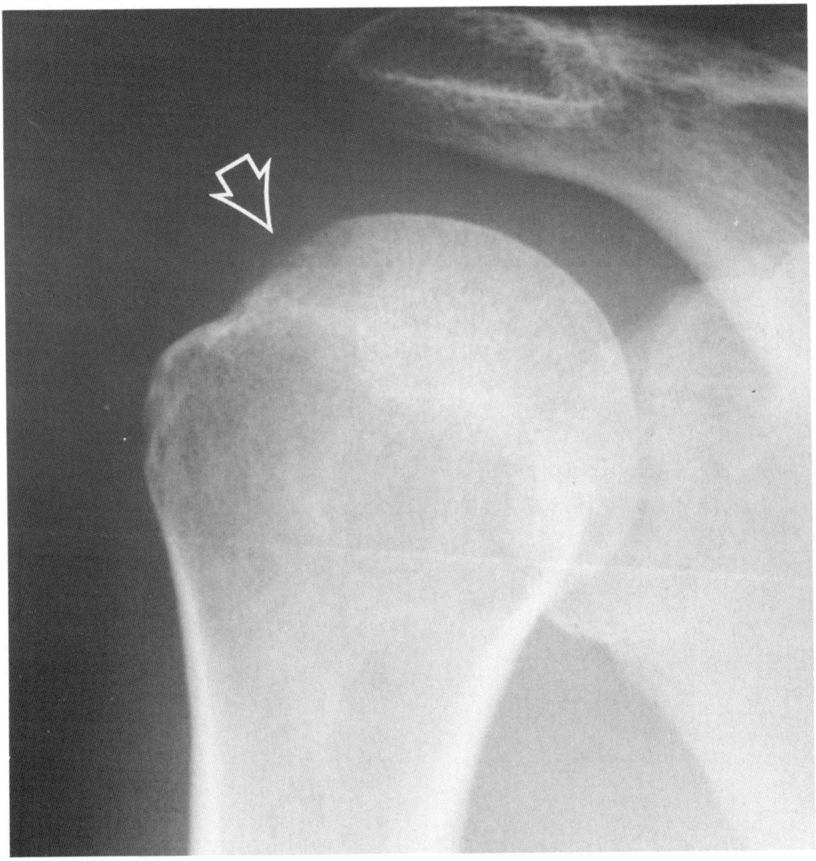

Figure 3-A

Tuberculosis arthritis. 43-year-old HIV-positive female drug abuser with tuberculous arthritis of the right shoulder. Original AP radiograph of the right shoulder shows mild osteopenia and erosion of the cortical margin of the lateral humeral head (open arrow).

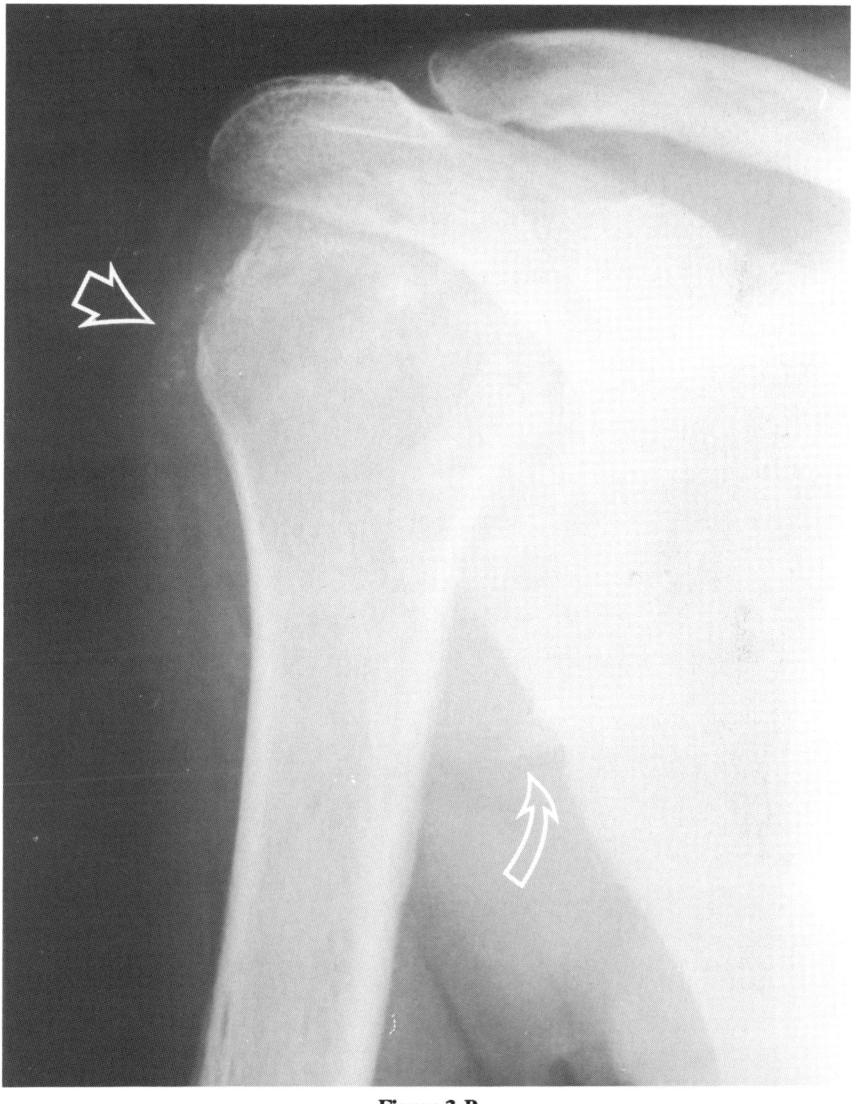

Figure 3-B

Plain radiograph of the right shoulder obtained one year later shows severe osteoporosis with resorption of the cortical margin of the glenohumeral joint, pathologic nondisplaced fracture with posterior dislocation of the shoulder, extensive soft tissue calcification (open arrows), high-riding of the humeral head, and atrophy of the rotator cuff.

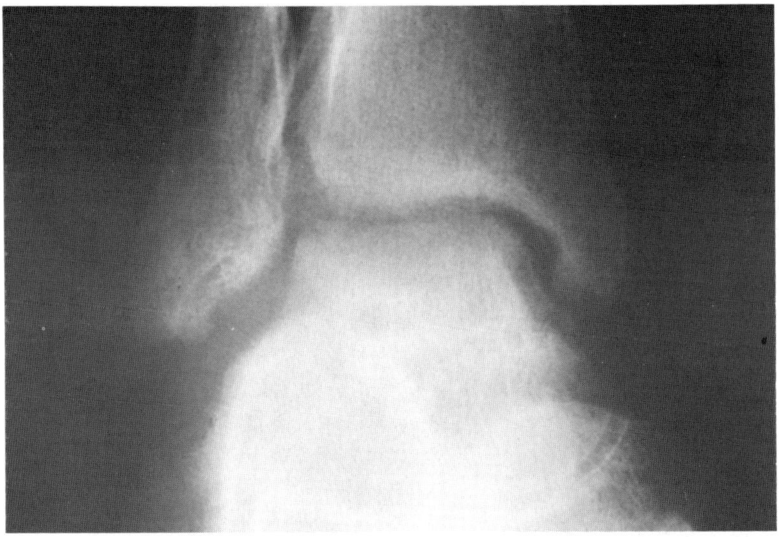

Figure 4-A

Tuberculosis arthritis. This is a 31-year-old HIV-positive female with tuberculous arthritis of the right ankle. AP (A) and lateral (B) plain radiographs of the right ankle show osteopenia, loss of cortices of the tibia and talus, narrowed joint spaces with erosive changes of the tibial plafond and dome of the talus, and erosive changes of the calcaneus. Note large joint effusion and soft tissue swelling.

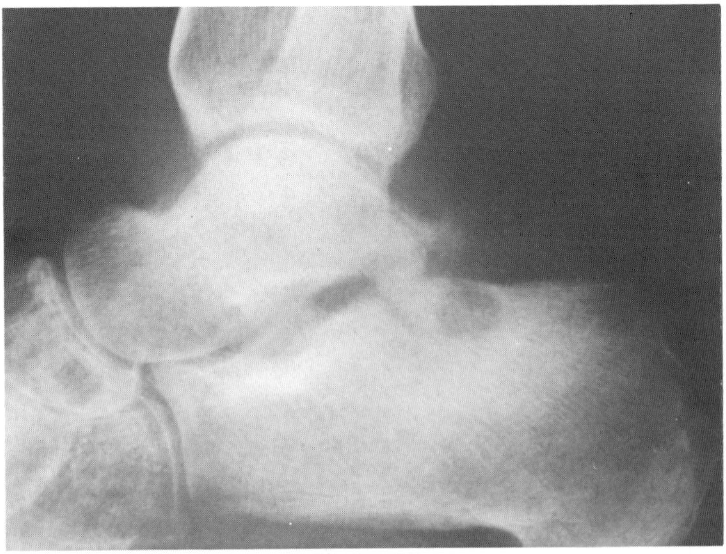

Figure 4-B

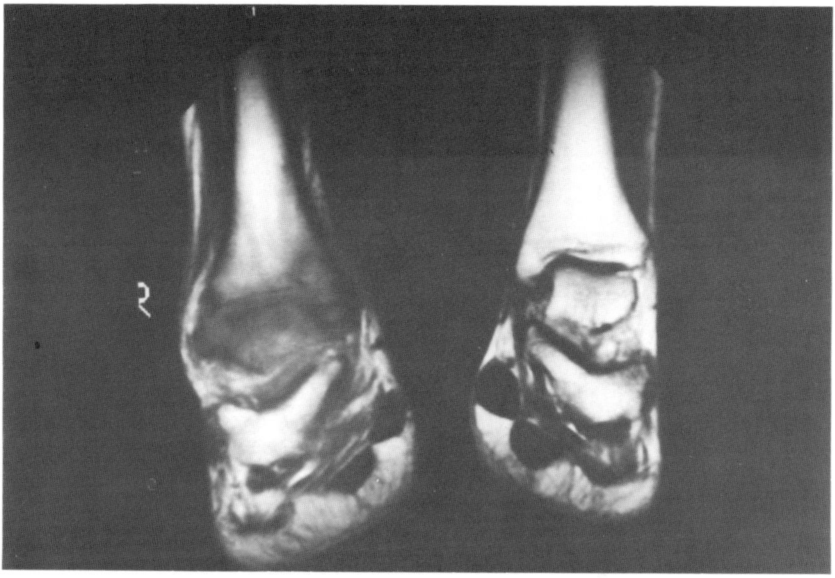

Figure 4-C

Coronal (C) and axial (D) T1-weighted images (TR 600, TE 26) show decreased signal intensity of the distal tibia, talus and calcaneus on the right side with adjacent soft tissue edema.

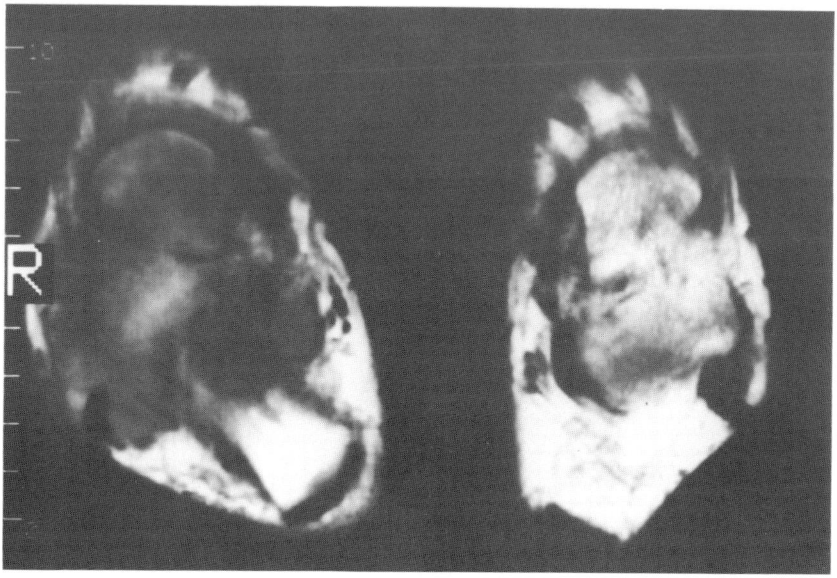

Figure 4-D

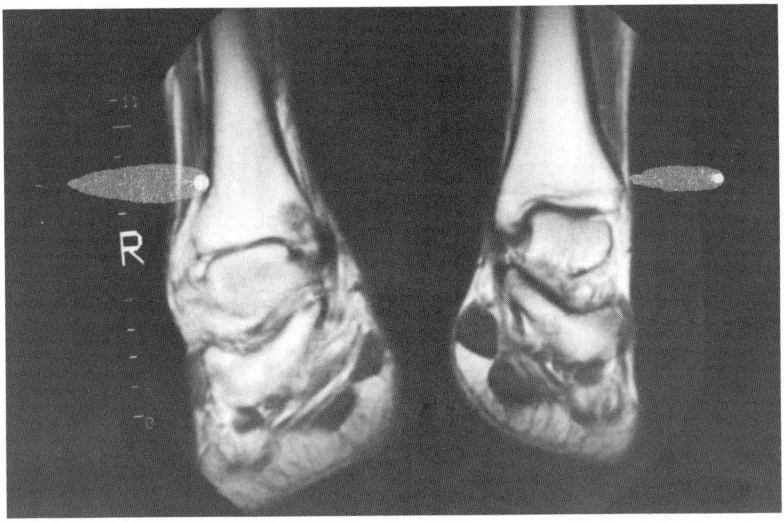

Figure 4-E

Coronal T1-weighted images (TR 600, TE 26) with intravenous gadolinium show enhancement of the inflamed synovium around the ankle joint, with enhancement of the marrow of the distal tibia and talus. Note medial malleolus remains relatively low in signal intensity and may be ischemic in relation to other areas.

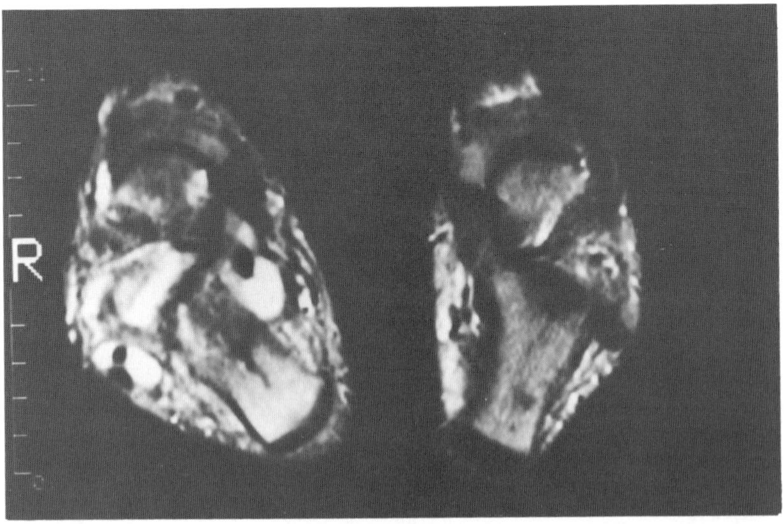

Figure 4-F

Axial T2-weighted images (TR 1800, TE 80) show edema of the soft tissues and fluid in the tendon sheath of the peroneal tendon and flexor hallucis longus. Note mixed (low and high) signal intensities in the talus and calcaneus on the right side.

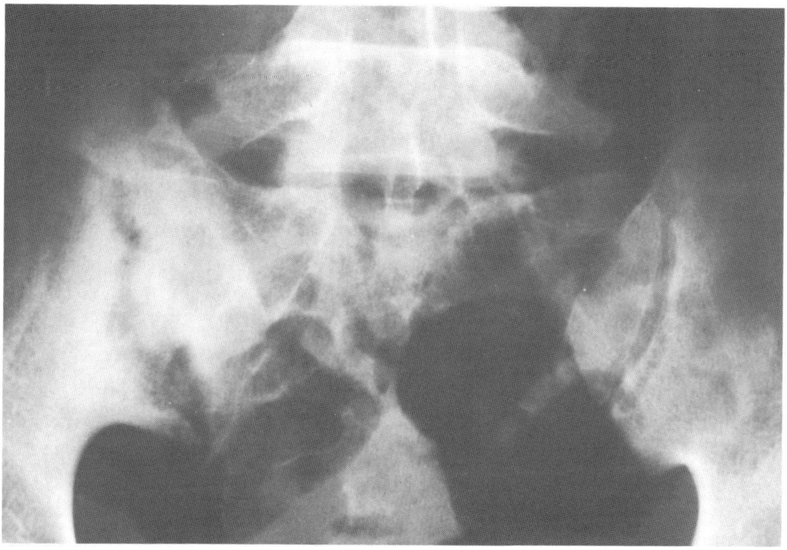

Figure 5-A

Tuberculosis sacroilitis. Right sacroiliitis in an HIV-positive patient with history of tuberculosis and syphilis. (From Vanarthos W, RadioGraphics 1992;12:731-749.) AP radiograph of the pelvis shows severe erosive as well as sclerotic changes in the right sacroiliac joint.

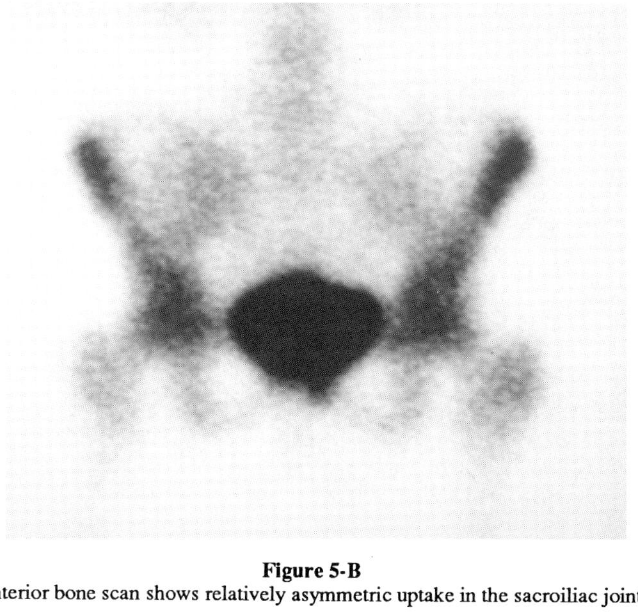

Figure 5-B

Anterior bone scan shows relatively asymmetric uptake in the sacroiliac joint.

REFERENCES

1. Barnes P, Bloch A, Davidson P, Snider D Jr. Tuberculosis in patients with human immunodeficiency virus infection. *NEJM* 324(23):1644-1650.
2. American Thoracic Society. Mycobacterioses and acquired immunodeficiency syndrome. *Am Rev Respir Dis* 1987;136:492-494.
3. Federle M (Guest editor). Radiology of the immunocompromised patient. *Rad Clin North Am* 30(3), May 1992.
4. Wolff M, Bitran J, Northland R, Levy I. Splenic abscesses due to mycobacterium tuberculosis in patients with AIDS. *Rev Infec Dis* 1991;13:373-375.
5. Pitchenik A, Rubinson H. The radiographic appearance of tuberculosis in patients with acquired immunodeficiency syndrome and pre-AIDS. *Am Rev Respir Dis* 1985;131:393-396.
6. Bargallo N, Nicolau C, Luburich P, Ayuso C, Cardenal C, Gimeno F. Intestinal tuberculosis in AIDS. *Gastrointest Radiol* 1992;17:115-118.
7. deSilva R, Stoopack P, Raufman J. Esophageal fistula associated with mycobacterial infection in patients at risk for AIDS. *Radiology* 1990;175:449-453.
8. Bishburg E, Sunderam G, Reichman LB, et al. Central nervous system tuberculosis with AIDS. *Ann Int Med* 1986;105:210-213.
9. Chapman M, Murray R, Stoker D. Tuberculosis of the bones and joints. *Semin Roentgenol* 1979;14(4).
10. Resnick D, Niwayama G. *Diagnosis of Bone and Joint Disorders,* 2nd ed. Philadelphia: W.B. Saunders, 1988.
11. Sharif H, et al. Granulomatous spinal infections: MR imaging. *Radiology* 1990; 177:101-107.
12. Steinbach LS, Tehranzadeh J, Fleckenstein JL, Vanarthos WJ, Pais MJ. Human immunodeficiency virus infection: musculoskeletal manifestations. *Radiology* 1993;186:833-838.
13. Vinetz JM, Rickman LS. Chronic arthritis due to mycobacterium avium complex infection in a patient with acquired immunodeficiency syndrome. *Arth Rheum* 1991 Oct;34(10):1339-1340.
14. Blumenthal DR, Zucker JR, Hawkins CC. Mycobacterium avium complex-induced septic arthritis and osteomyelitis in a patient with the acquired immunodeficiency syndrome (Letter). *Arth Rheum* 1990 May;33(5):757-758.
15. Kristjansson M, Bieluch VM, Byeff PD. Mycobacterium haemophilum infection in immunocompromised patients: case report and review of the literature. *Rev Infect Dis* 1991 Sep-Oct;13(5):906-910.

16. Males BM, West TE, Bartholomew WR. Mycobacterium haemophilum infection in a patient with acquired immunodeficiency syndrome. J *Clin Microbiol* 1987 Jan; 25(1):186-190.
17. Pouchot J, Vinceneux P, Barge J, Laparre F, Boussougant Y, Michon C. Tuberculous polymyositis in HIV infection (Letter). *Am J Med* 1990 Aug;89(2):250-251.

CHAPTER 4:

MUSCULAR MANIFESTATIONS IN THE ACQUIRED IMMUNODEFICIENCY SYNDROME (AIDS)

James L. Fleckenstein, M.D.

INTRODUCTION

Weakness is a common feature of AIDS that is often assumed to result from any number of common and uncommon AIDS-related central nervous system complications [1-9]. This fact contributes to the difficulty in diagnosing treatable causes of weakness that are due to disorders of the peripheral nervous system and/or skeletal muscle. A broad variety of pathological alterations of muscle have been reported in both biopsy [8,10] and autopsy series [11] of patients with AIDS. In these series, the range of pathological conditions spanned nonspecific findings such as angulated fibers and fiber atrophy, and specific etiologies such as *Mycobacterial avium intracellulare* myositis and *Cryptococcus neoformans* myositis [11]. Because diagnostic imaging techniques have the ability to detect and characterize lesions of muscles, imaging modalities may be helpful to clinicians in evaluating muscle lesions of unclear etiology in AIDS patients.

Muscle abnormalities in AIDS which can be expected to be visible on some imaging studies include drug-related myopathies [12-18], immune-mediated inflammatory myopathies (e.g. polymyositis) [1,6,11,19-22], infectious myositides [1,11,23-26], lymphedema [23], denervation due to peripheral neuropathies [4,5,10,11,27-32], and other myopathies [11,33,34]. This chapter will review the spectrum of diseases that may affect muscle in AIDS patients and will summarize the available literature regarding imaging techniques in these conditions.

Drug-related Myopathy

A myopathy is recognized in AIDS patients that is induced by the commonly prescribed antiviral drug, zidovudine (also referred to as azidothymidine)

[12-18]. Histopathology in such cases has revealed "ragged red" fibers, indicative of abnormal mitochondria, and paracrystalline inclusions [13]. Interestingly, an associated inflammatory myopathy, indistinguishable from polymyositis in non-HIV patients, is observed in the patients with drug-related mitochondrial alterations. Cessation of treatment with zidovudine is associated with marked histological and clinical improvement. Although there are no reported cases of proven AZT-related myopathy in the imaging literature, one could speculate that imaging modalities would reveal findings typical of mitochondrial myopathy (selective deterioration of the sartorius and gracilis) [35] and/or polymyositis (selective sparing of the sartorius and gracilis) [36].

Myositides

The incidence of bacteremia and fungemia in AIDS has been observed to be increased compared to that of the general population [37]. This likely contributes to the observed increased incidence of bacterial, and other, myositides in AIDS.

Infectious myositis in AIDS may be caused by a host of organisms including bacteria, fungi, and parasites [8,11,34,38,39]. Viral myositis, caused by HIV itself, appears to be extremely rare, if it exists at all[8], although myositis due to co-infection with Human T-Cell Leukemia Virus Type 1 (HTLV-1) in a patient with AIDS has been reported [22]. Idiopathic inflammatory myopathy, i.e. polymyositis, an autoimmune disorder, also occurs in AIDS and may precede onset of signs and symptoms of AIDS in the HIV+ patient [1,19,37,40].

Pyogenic Bacterial Myositis (Pyomyositis)

Although rare in the United States, pyogenic bacterial myositis (pyomyositis) is very common in the tropics [41]. It is usually caused by *Staphylococus aureus* and is typically diagnosed in otherwise healthy males. However, outside of the tropics, pyogenic myositis tends to occur in patients who are malnourished or are immunodeficient for other reasons [21,24,38,40,42-49]. A high index of suspicion is required because clinical signs of inflammation are mild in the early stages; fever and leukocytosis are low grade, if present, and physical examination is characterized by a nonspecific "wooden" stiffness without fluctuance. In the more advanced stages, the skeletal muscle may be almost totally destroyed and replaced by pus [41].

Recognition of bacterial myositis in AIDS is important because it represents a readily curable condition in AIDS that may be fatal if not recognized. A few case reports have documented the utility of scintigraphy to detect pyomyositis in AIDS and other immunocompromised states. These include ^{67}Gallium [38,40,46,50,51], ^{111}Indium-tagged white blood cells [38], and ^{99m}Technetium [38,40,43,46] bone scans. By virtue of ^{67}Gallium or ^{111}Indium nuclide accumulation, foci of inflammation can be roughly localized to the muscles. Using ^{99m}Tc phosphates, pyomyositis is typically inapparent when only a delayed scan is performed but is detectible if immediate and "blood pool" scintigrams are obtained, due to hyperemia associated with the inflammatory process [38,40,43,46]. This is important since if only a delayed study is performed, pyomyositis may go undiagnosed. It is further noteworthy that Kaposi's sarcoma of the muscle may share the appearance of pyomyositis on 3-phase ^{99m}Tc bone scans (see Fig. 6). Also, other pathologic conditions of muscle, such as myositis ossificans [50] or polymyositis [21], may concentrate radionuclide tracers in the muscles of AIDS patients.

Ultrasound and CT may also be useful to localize and characterize pyomyositis, although both have limitations. At ultrasound, echointensity may be increased or decreased with respect to normal muscle, depending on whether the tissue is phlegmonous or liquefied [38,43,48]. CT may be helpful to determine if drainable fluid is present [38,42,46,52,57], but is limited by beam-hardening artifacts obscuring soft tissues and by its inherently poor sensitivity to muscle edema. On MRI, bacterial myositis frequently demonstrates a peculiar appearance, characterized on T1-weighted images by a rim of high signal intensity around a central region isointense to normal muscle (Fig. 1). While the

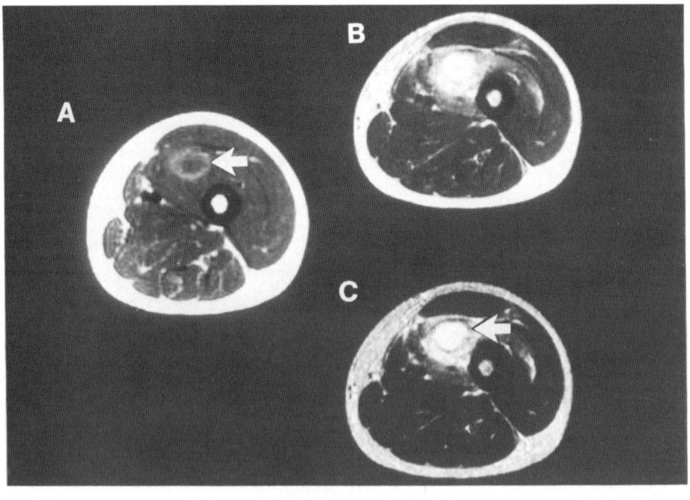

Figure 1-A, B & C

Pyogenic bacterial myositis (pyomyositis) in AIDS. An hyperintense rim sign is visible in the left vastus medialis muscle on a T1-weighted MR sequence (500/30) (arrow, A); note a closely associated hypointense band on T2-weighted MR sequence (2000/90) (arrow, C). The proton density (2000/30) (B) and T2-weighted (2000/90) (C) MR images show a central focus of extremely high signal intensity (light bulb sign), corresponding to subsequently drained pus. Muscle edema surrounds the central portion in (B) and (C). Cultures of aspirated fluid yielded *Staphylococcus aureus*.

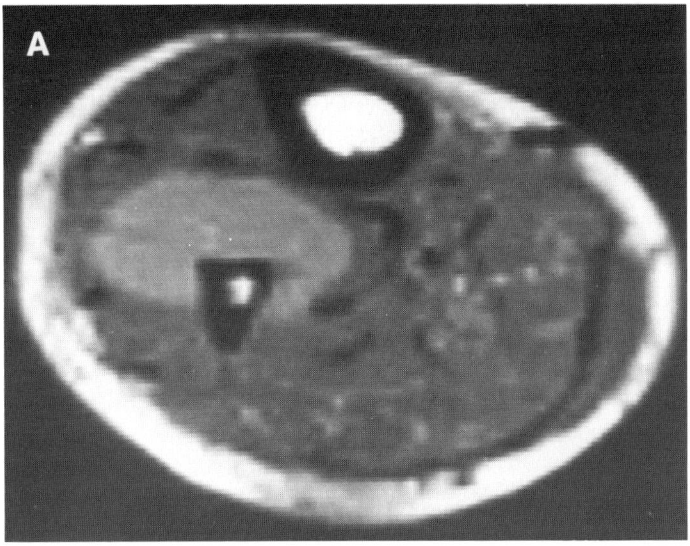

Figure 2-A

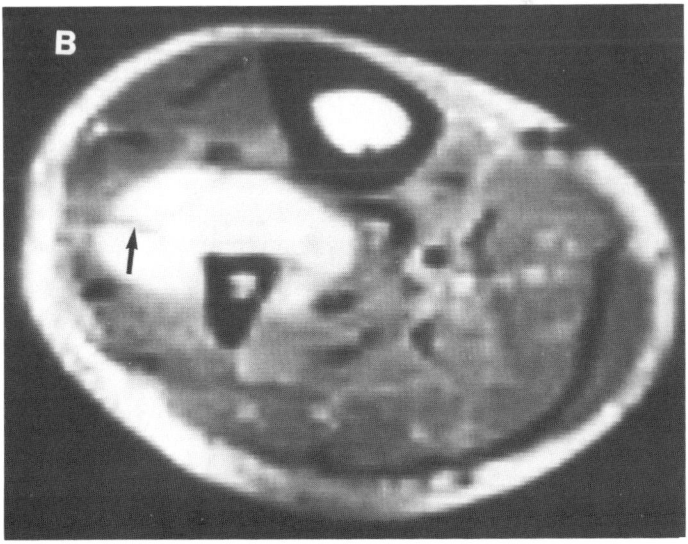

Figure 2-B

Multifocal pyogenic bacterial myositis in AIDS. Signal intensity surrounding the fibula is increased compared to muscle on T1-weighted (500/30) (A) and T2-weighted (2000/60) (B) MR images. The process crosses fascial boundaries (e.g. arrow, B). Similar findings were present in a muscle abscess in the contralateral limb. Aspiration of leg lesions yielded frank pus, which cultured positive for *Staphylococcus aureus*. (From Fleckenstein JL: *Radiology* 1991;179:653-658).

physical basis of this MRI finding has not been definitively identified, paramagnetic material is a possibility. Potential etiologies include methemoglobin from subacute bleeding, bacterial or macrophage sequestration of iron, and/or the occurrence of free radicals in the rim. Associated rims of decreased signal intensity on T2-weighted images might then be due to conglomerated (superparamagnetic) iron such as present in hemosiderin. Fibrous tissue deposition within the "wall" of the abscess could also contribute to the hypointense appearance on T2-weighted images [23,47].

Additional T1-weighted MRI appearances of drainable pus include isointensity or homogeneously increased signal intensity with respect to normal muscle but without an associated hyperintense rim (Fig. 2) [23]. Regardless of the appearance of abscesses on T1-weighted images, central portions of the abscesses show extremely increased signal intensity on Short-tau Inversion-Recovery (STIR) and T2-weighted images (Figs. 1,2). On these images, more diffuse and milder signal intensity changes may become visible in muscle peripheral to the abscess. The ability to use MRI to suggest the presence of drainable fluid may thus enhance clinical management of AIDS patients. It is also noteworthy that muscle abscesses are frequently multiple, a finding present in 30% of bacterial myositis [41]. MRI may be useful for evaluating potential additional lesions due to its high sensitivity, although whole-body scintigraphic studies such as ^{111}Indium-tagged white blood cell examination may be more practical for screening the entire body for additional lesions. Since the muscle-tendon junction may be the site of abscess formation, the ability of MRI to accurately delineate this structure can facilitate localization of such lesions (Fig. 3).

Yuh, et al, reporting on MRI findings in two cases of bacterial myositis without AIDS, emphasized the important differential diagnosis of bacterial myositis and cellulitis, suggesting that disproportionate involvement of the muscles in comparison to subcutaneous tissue favored the diagnosis of bacterial myositis [49]. However, this distinction is obscured by the observation that edematous subcutaneous tissue is also present in the situation of lymphedema, a condition that occurs in AIDS when lymphatic obstruction results from either disseminated lymphoma or Kaposi's sarcoma (see below) [23]. Hence, the appearance of subcutaneous edema is not specific for cellulitis and careful clinical correlation is necessary so that a relatively benign diagnosis (cellulitis) is not assumed to be present when a more ominous disease is present.

Mycobacterial Myositis

Mycobacterial infection is very common in AIDS patients and, in fact, mycobacteria constitute the most common cause of sepsis in AIDS [37]. Hence,

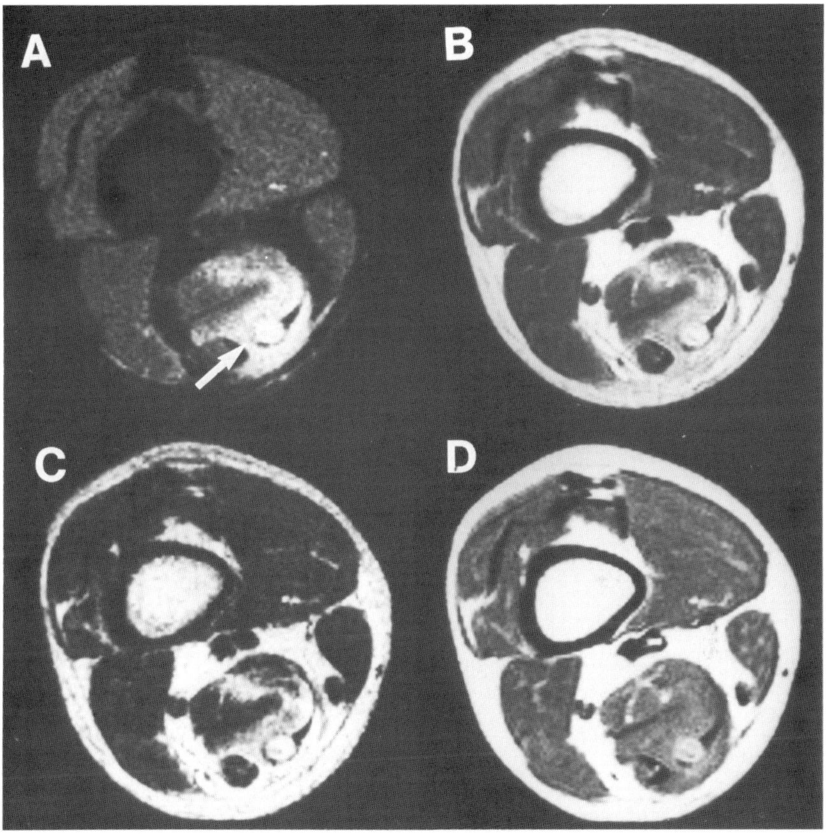

Figure 3

Tendon abscess in AIDS. A focal area of increased signal intensity is seen in the tendon of the semimembranosus on STIR (1500/30/100, TR/TE/TI)(arrow, A), proton density (2000/30) (B), T2-weighted (2000/90) (C), and T1-weighted (500/30) (D) MR images. Associated edema-like signal intensity changes of the adjacent muscle are also observed. Blood cultures grew group B *Streptococcus pyogenes* and appropriate antibiotic treatment was instituted. Three months later, a repeat MRI documented complete resolution of the lesion (not shown). (From Fleckenstein JL: *Radiology* 1991;179:653-58.)

it is not surprising that mycobacterial myositis has been reported in AIDS [11,23]. To date, the imaging findings in this condition have not been reported. However, Figure 4 shows a patient with sacroiliitis and a swollen forearm. The forearm lesion, proven at autopsy to be due to mycobacterial myositis, was evident on 3-phase bone scintigraphy, ^{111}Indium-labeled leukocyte study, and on MRI. The features were nonspecific, however, and cannot be distinguished from pyogenic infection.

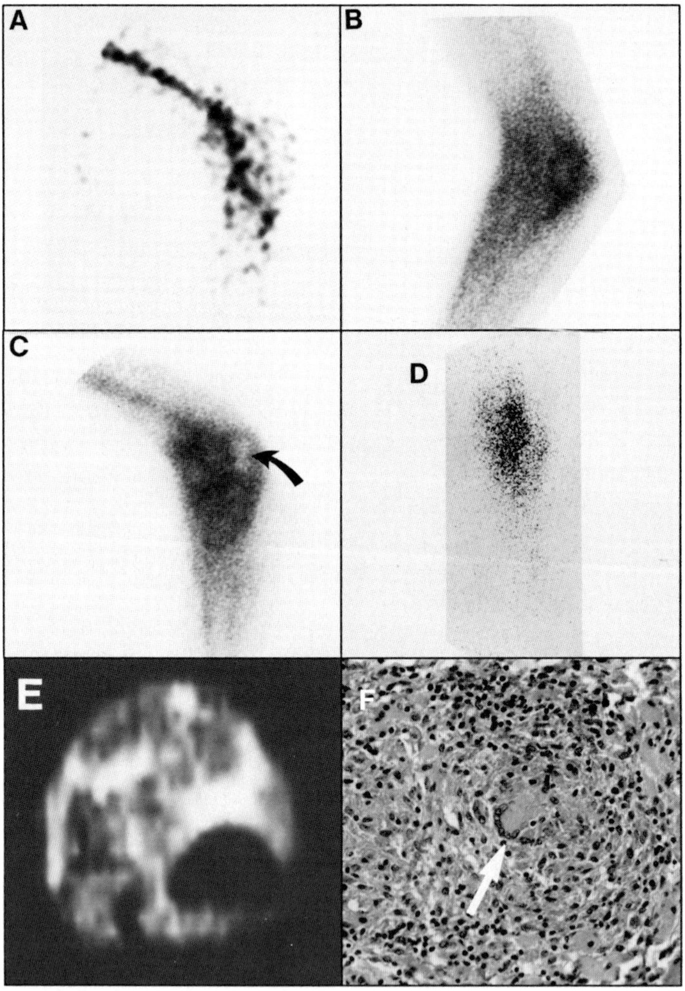

Figure 4-A, B, C, D, E, & F

Mycobacterial myositis. This patient presented with tuberculous sacroiliitis and a swollen painful forearm. Triple-phase bone scan of the elbow reveals increased tracer delivery to the soft tissues near the elbow, as shown on immediate (A) and blood pool (B) scintigrams. After a 3 hour delay, increased tracer activity is seen adjacent to a focal photopenic area (arrow, C). Autologously labeled ^{111}Indium white cells accumulate in the same region 24 hours after injection (D). Five days prior to death, agitation limited the MRI examination to a low spatial resolution, 1 minute STIR (1500/30/95, TR/TE/TI, E) sequence of the distal arm. Even at low resolution, the STIR image reveals markedly increased signal intensity heterogeneously distributed in the muscles. Note that the fat is normally suppressed in the humeral shaft, indicating absence of bone marrow involvement. Postmortem muscle specimen from this region shows multinucleated giant cells (arrow, F). Muscle culture was positive for *Mycobacterium tuberculosis*.

Fungal and Parasitic Myositis

To the author's knowledge, no cases of fungal or parasitic myositis have been reported using imaging studies, despite the fact that such cases have been proven using histopathological means [11,24].

Autoimmune Myositis (Polymyositis)

Idiopathic inflammatory myositis (polymyositis) is a well-recognized cause of muscular weakness and serum creatine kinase elevation in HIV-infected patients, occurring in some patients before the classical signs of AIDS develop [4]. Interestingly, polymyositis occurs in 50% of primates with experimentally-induced AIDS [53]. Recently, attention has been focused on the use of MRI to detect edematous muscles of patients without AIDS prior to biopsy and in grading the severity of disease and the response to therapy [39]. A recent case of an HIV+ patient who presented with proximal muscle weakness lead to an MRI study that documented edematous changes in the posterior leg muscles (Fig. 5). Biopsy performed in the MRI suite confirmed the presence of lymphocyte infiltration in the muscle, establishing the diagnosis of polymyositis. The case also demonstrates that although polymyositis is classically considered to present with proximal muscle weakness, the more distal muscles are also affected (47).

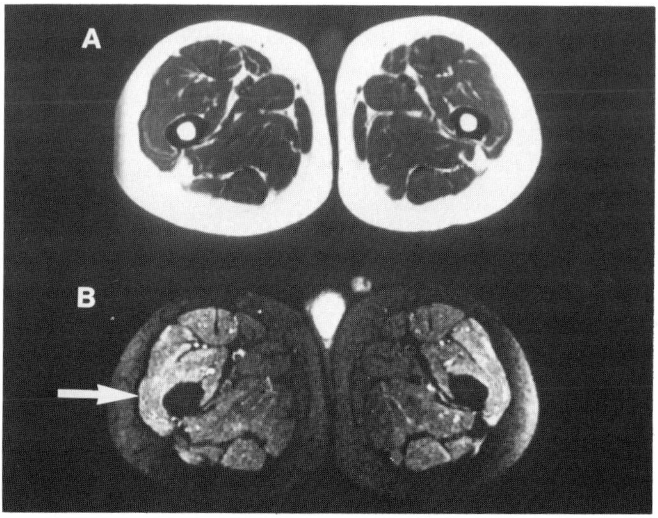

Figure 5-A & B.

HIV-associated idiopathic myopathy (polymyositis). T1-weighted (500/30) (A) and STIR (1500/30/100, TR/TE/TI) (B) MR images of the proximal thighs show minimal alterations, primarily restricted to mild edema-like changes of the vastus lateralis (arrow, B).

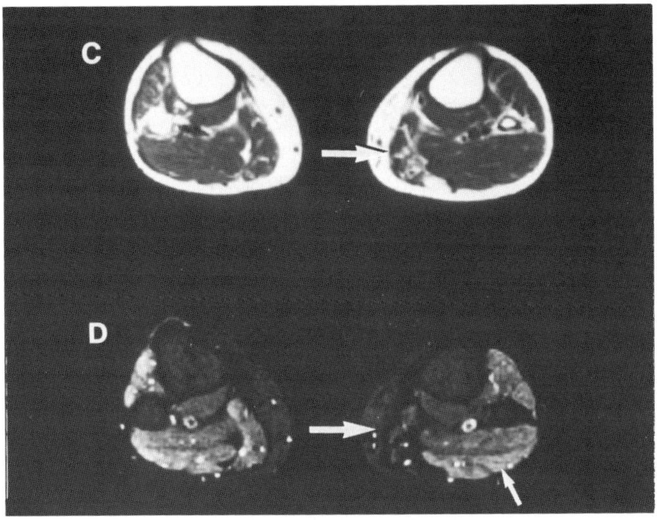

Figure 5-C & D

T1-weighted (500/30) (C) and STIR (D) images of the proximal legs show more marked abnormalities, characterized by mild fatty infiltration, evident by high signal intensity in the left medial gastrocnemius (arrow, C) and by hypointensity on the fat-suppressed STIR sequence (1500/30/100, TR/TE/TI) (arrow, D). The more "active" location of inflammation is suggested by edema-like changes, i.e. STIR hyperintensity. The relatively hyperintense left lateral gastrocnemius muscle (small arrow, D) was selected for biopsy, yielding infiltrating lymphocytes, securing the diagnosis of polymyositis.

Neurogenic Muscle Disease in AIDS

Peripheral neuropathy is common in AIDS, being suspected in up to 40% of AIDS patients [4,10,11,27-29,31,32]. Biopsy and autopsy studies have shown an inflammatory neuropathy with a variable component of demyelination and axonal loss. Evidence of direct nerve infection by HIV is scant, although cytomegalovirus has been demonstrated in multiple cases to be a direct cause of polyradiculopathy [4,10,11,27-29,31,32]. Although no imaging study of muscle disease related to denervation in AIDS has been reported, the high sensitivity of MRI in detecting edema-like muscle changes caused by denervation would predict that denervation may cause an appearance of muscle similar to polymyositis [54]. Hence, denervation should be remembered as a differential diagnostic possibility in the patient whose MRI study shows edema-like changes restricted to the muscles. It remains to be established whether disuse atrophy, as one would expect in the wasting syndrome of AIDS, is a cause of similar changes on MRI of muscle.

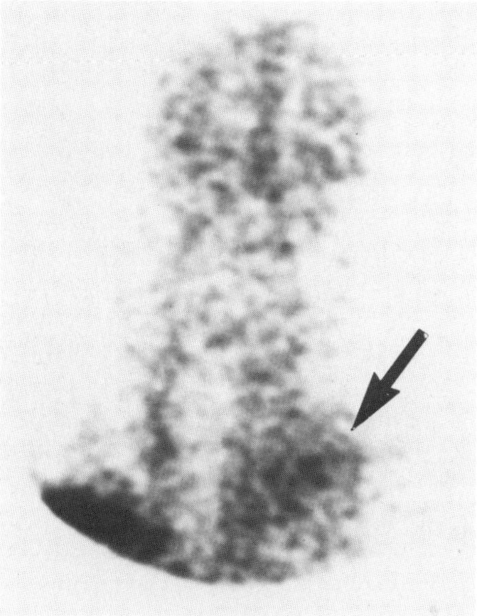

Figure 6-A

Kaposi's sarcoma of muscle. The patient presented with a painful swelling in the left neck. Lymphoma was suspected clinically. Triple-phase bone scan reveals increased tracer delivery to the area (arrows), as shown on immediate (A) and blood pool (B) scintigrams.

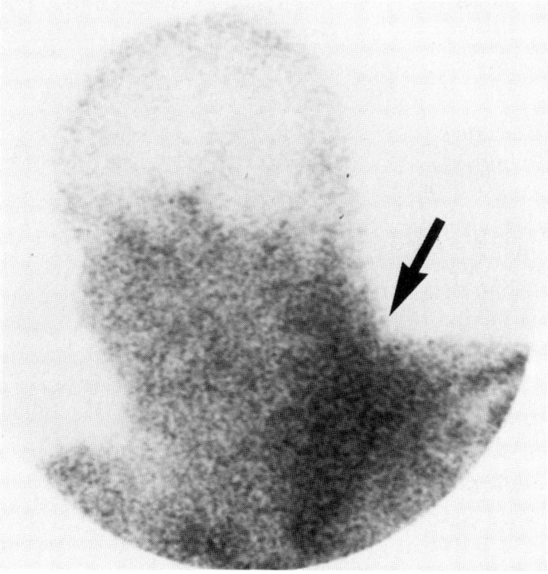

Figure 6-B

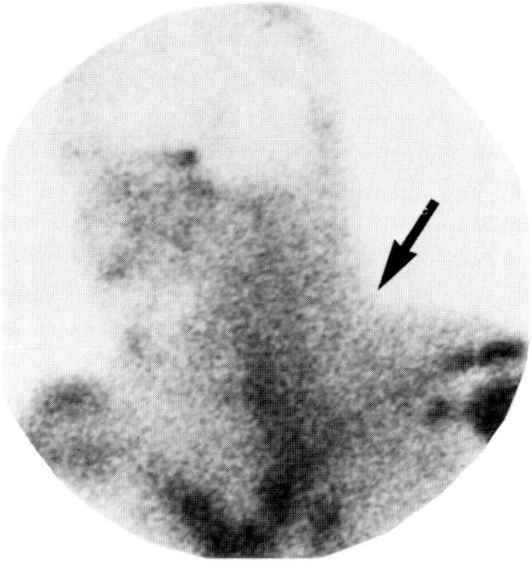

Figure 6-C

After a 3-hour delay, no abnormality of tracer accumulation is seen.

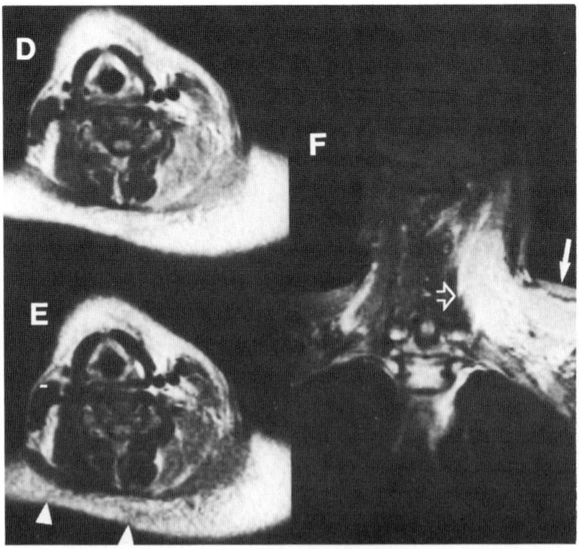

Figure 6-D, E & F

Axial proton density (2000/30)(D) and T1-weighted (500/30) (E) MR images show increased muscle signal intensity compared to normal muscle on the left with reticulated signal intensity alteration of the subcutaneous tissues being detectible on the T1-weighted (500/30) MR image (arrowheads, E). Coronal STIR (1500/30/100) image shows the longitudinal extent of the muscle involvement (arrowhead, F). Hyperintensity of the subcutaneous fat on STIR indicates edema-like changes (arrow, F).

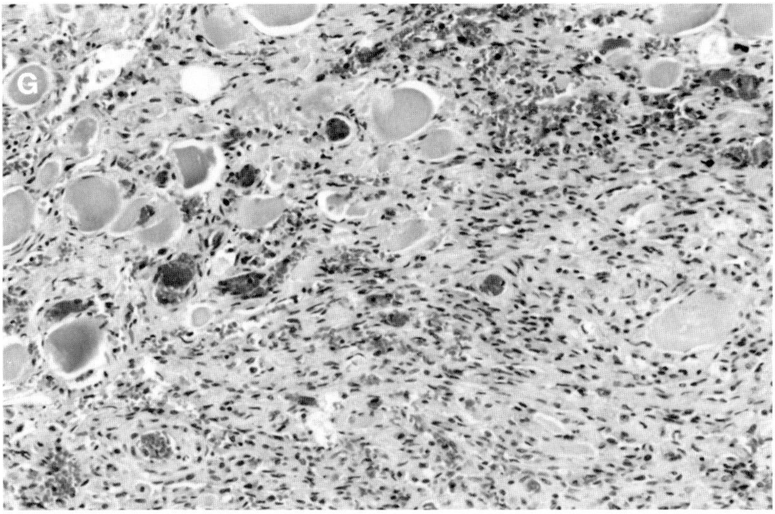

Figure 6-G

Postmortem specimen shows typical findings of Kaposi's sarcoma, including spindle-shaped cells in a hypervascular stroma (G).

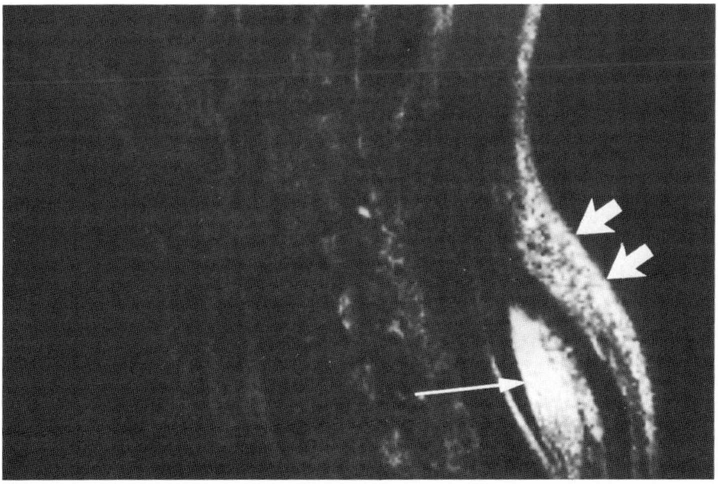

Figure 6-H

A sagittal T2-weighted (2000/120) MR image of the neck in a second patient shows hyperintense muscle (arrow, H) and abnormal streaky changes to the subcutaneous fat (arrowheads), findings suggestive of Kaposi's sarcoma.

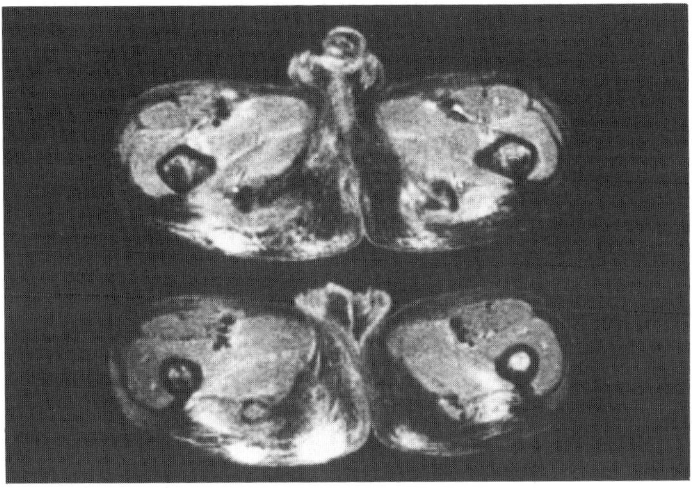

Figure 7

Carbunculosis in an AIDS patient. Contiguous 1 cm STIR images (1500/30/100, TR/TE/TI) of the affected region show foci of markedly increased signal intensity, not only in the subcutaneous fat but also in the gluteus and adductor muscles, indicating edematous change of both types of soft tissue.

Muscle Edema in the Setting of Edematous Subcutaneous Tissues

One study employed MRI to evaluate the extremities of patients with AIDS and observed a pattern of abnormality which appeared distinct from that described for myositis [23]. Whereas in myositis, edema-like changes were primarily restricted to the muscles themselves, in the second pattern both the subcutaneous tissues and the muscles showed edema-like alterations. In one case, Kaposi's Sarcoma was found (Fig. 6) while in another case infection was found (Fig. 7). In the others there was no support for cellulitis as the cause for the edematous subcutaneous tissues (Figs. 8-10), although one patient was treated for a protracted period for that diagnosis. In that patient (Fig. 8), biopsy of a superficial forearm nodule yielded lymphoma and the subcutaneous edema was presumed secondary to lymphatic obstruction due to lymphoma. Another case was shown to be due to lymphatic obstruction due to Kaposi's sarcoma [23]. In the author's experience, this pattern of edema in the muscles and subcutaneous tissues is at least as frequent as isolated muscle alterations but the etiology is frequently more difficult to prove. In a series of 7 patients with such a pattern, vascular imaging studies excluded venous thrombosis as the etiology for the alterations. This is important because the only series comparing the MRI appearance of extremity edema due to venous thrombosis (phlebedema) to that of lymphedema in patients without AIDS reported that muscles tend to be normal

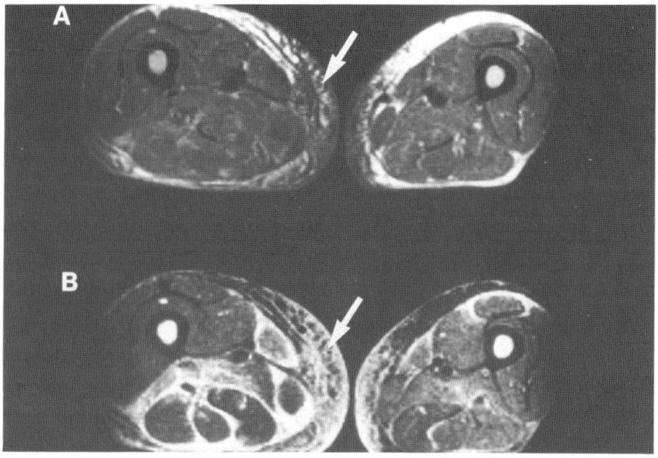

Figure 8-A & B

Lymphoma-associated lymphedema in AIDS. Axial T1-weighted (500/30) MR image of the thighs (A) shows skin thickening, subcutaneous tissue expansion and a "honeycomb" pattern of low signal intensity streaks in the subcutaneous tissue (arrow, A). STIR image at the same level (1500/30/100, TR/TE/TI) (B) shows abnormally increased signal intensity in the subcutaneous fat (arrow) and a variable degree of increased signal intensity in and around some thigh muscles. Axial T1-weighted (500/30) MR image of the forearms, was centered on a palpable mass (arrow, C), subsequently biopsied and found to contain high-grade lymphoma. STIR image at the same level (1500/30/100, TR/TE/TI) (D) shows increased signal intensity in the subcutaneous and intermuscular perifascial regions. (From Fleckenstein JL: *Radiology* 1991;179:653-658.)

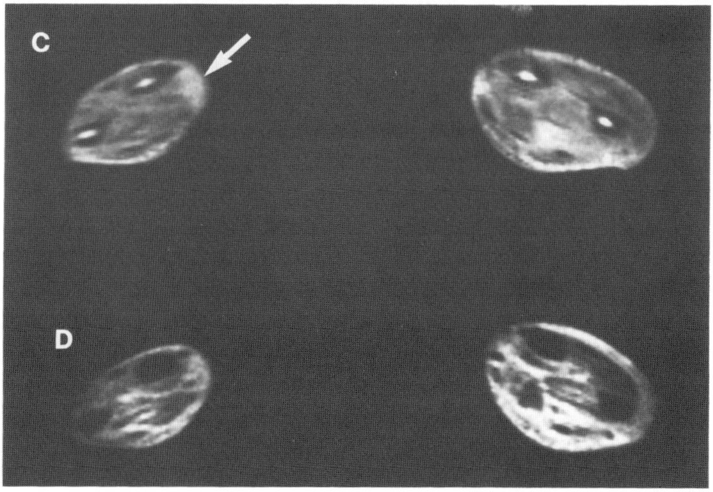

Figure 8-C & D

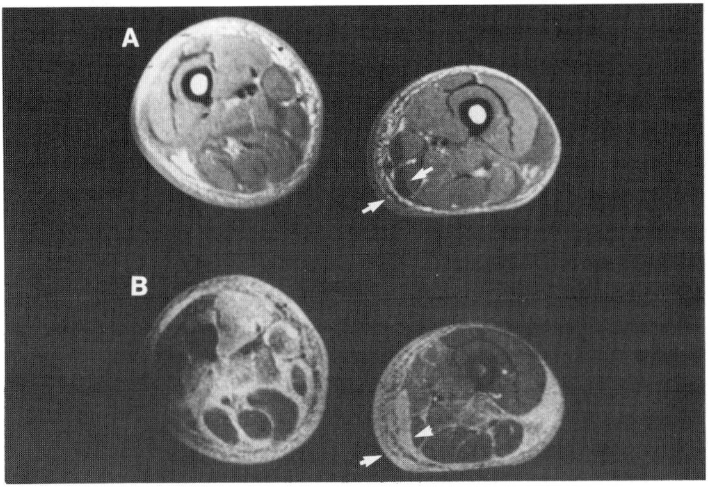

Figure 9-A & B

Lymphedema pattern in AIDS patient with disseminated Kaposi's sarcoma and slowly progressive, asymmetric "brawny edema" of the lower extremities. T1-weighted MR images of the thighs (500/30) (A) show skin thickening, subcutaneous "honeycomb" appearance and fluid collections (between arrows). While subcutaneous tissue (fat) is usually suppressed using the STIR sequence (1500/30/100, TR/TE/TI), the fat is abnormally hyperintense on this image (between arrows, B). Muscle edema is easily seen upon inspection of the right thigh in the STIR image.

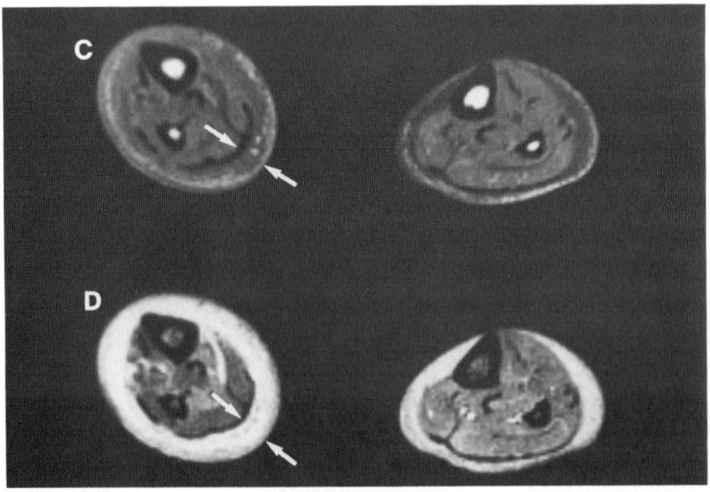

Figure 9-C & D

Axial images of the legs show abnormal subcutaneous hypointensity using a Tl-weighted MR sequence (500/30) (C) and markedly increased signal intensity using the STIR sequence (D). Note asymmetric enlargement of the edematous subcutaneous tissue (between arrows, C,D).

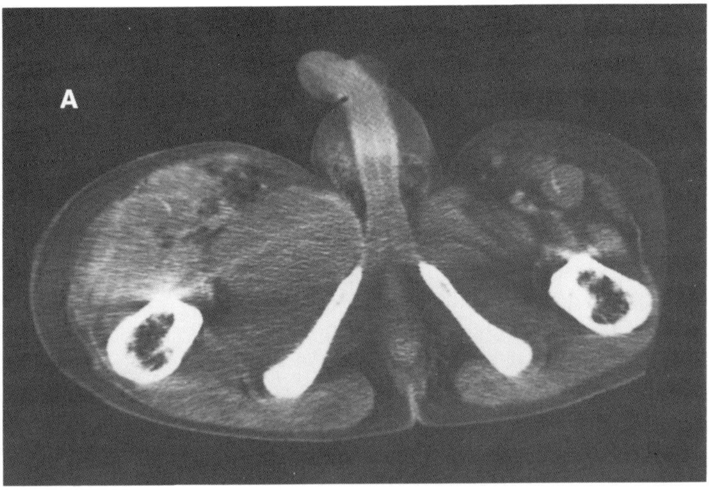

Figure 10-A

Lymphedema pattern in AIDS. Unenhanced CT scan of the lower pelvis and proximal thighs shows swelling of the right thigh and abnormally dense subcutaneous fat (A).

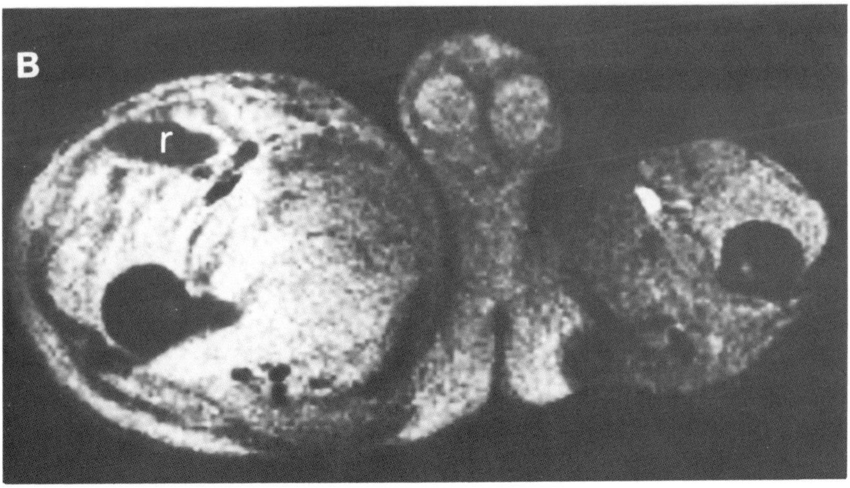

Figure 10-B

STIR (1500/30/100, TR/TE/TI) (B) shows to better advantage the edema in the subcutaneous fat on the right as well as apparent sparing of only the rectus femoris muscle (r), with all other right-sided muscles being markedly infiltrated by high signal intensity material. It also shows a relative lack of involvement of left thigh muscles and subcutaneous fat. A venogram excluded deep venous thrombosis. Blindly performed aspiration of swollen tissues yielded only negative cultures and puncture sites oozed serous fluid. The patient died without a diagnosis but the case illustrates the superior depiction of soft tissue pathology using MRI compared to CT.

in lymphedema and edematous and swollen in phlebedema [55,56]. That conclusion is consistent with data from the CT literature [57], but it should be noted that CT is extremely limited in evaluating muscle edema and the MRI study did not use the highly sensitive STIR sequence to search for muscle edema. Also, it remains possible that in AIDS, the rapidity with which lymph vessels become engorged may affect the tendency to produce lymphatic stasis in muscles, visible by MRI.

CONCLUSIONS

This chapter has dealt primarily with muscle lesions that have been imaged either by the author or as reported in the literature. Given the broad spectrum of muscle diseases that occur in AIDS, it is doubtless that additional diseases could be detected by the various imaging modalities. Nemaline rods, for example, have been reported to occur in muscles of AIDS patients [33]. This myopathic finding may be visible in AIDS patients by a variety of imaging techniques since ultrasound, CT and MRI findings in such a condition have been reported in a non-AIDS patient [58]. The differential diagnosis of muscle disease that may be encountered by imaging studies in AIDS is therefore likely more exhaustive than that reported here. Hence, the "gold standard" for abnormal muscles in AIDS must remain the muscle biopsy. The imaging features should be used as a guide for definitive diagnostic tests including biopsy and for the follow-up of muscle lesions found in this group of patients.

REFERENCES

1. Berman A, Espinoza L, Diaz J, Aguilar J, Rolando T, Vasey F, Germain B, Lockey R. Rheumatic manifestations of human immunodeficiency virus infection. *Am J Med* 1988;85:59-64.
2. Britton C, Miller J. Neurologic complications in the acquired immunodeficiency syndrome (AIDS). *Neurol Clin* 1984;2:315-339.
3. Dalakas M. Neuromuscular complications of AIDS. *Muscle Nerve* 1986;9:92.
4. Dalakas M, Illa I, Pezeshkpour G, et al. Neuromuscular diseases associated with human immunodeficiency virus infection. *Ann Neurol* 1988(Suppl):S38-S48.
5. Gabuzda D, Hirsch M. Neurologic manifestations of infection with human immunodeficiency virus. Clinical features and pathogenesis. *Ann Intern Med* 1987;107:383-391.
6. Kaye B. Rheumatologic manifestations of infection with human immunodeficiencyvirus (HIV). *Ann Intern Med* 1989;111:158-167.
7. Lange D, Britton C, Younger D, Hays A. The neuromuscular manifestations of human immunodeficiency virus infections. *Arch Neurol* 1988;45:1084-1088.

8. Simpson D, Bender A. HIV-associated myopathy: analysis of 11 patients. *Ann Neurol* 1988;24:79-84.
9. Simpson D, Bender A, Farraye J, Mendelson S, Wolfe D. HIV wasting syndrome may represent a treatable myopathy. *Neurology* 1990;40:535-538.
10. Gabbai A, Schmidt B, Castelo A, Oliveira A, Lima J. Muscle biopsy in AIDS and ARC: analysis of 50 patients. *Muscle Nerve* 1990;13:541-544.
11. Wrzolek M, Sher J, Kozlowski P, Rao C. Skeletal muscle pathology in AIDS: an autopsy study. *Muscle Nerve* 1990;13:508-515.
12. Bessen L, Greene J, Louie E, Seitzman P, Weinberg H. Severe polymyositis-like syndrome associated with zidovudine therapy of AIDS and ARC (letter). *NEJM* 1988;318:708.
13. Dalakas M, Illa I, Pezeshkpour G, et al. Mitochondrial myopathy caused by long term zidovudine therapy. *NEJM* 1990;322:1098-1105.
14. Gertner E, Thurn J, Williams D, Simpson M, Balfour H, Rhame F, Henry K. Zidovudine-associated myopathy. *Am J Med* 1989;86:814-818.
15. Gonard D, Henry K, Guiloff R. Necrotising myopathy and zidovudine (letter). *Lancet* 1988;1:1050-1051.
16. Gorard D, Henry K, Guiloff R. Necrotising myopathy and zidovudine. *Lancet* 1988;1050.
17. Helbert M, Fletcher T, Peddle B, Harris J, Pinching A. Zidovudine-associated myopathy. *Lancet* 1988;ii:689-690.
18. Panegyres P, Tan N, Kakules B, Armstrong J, Hollingsworth P. Necrotising myopathy and zidovudine. *Lancet* 1988;I:1050-1051.
19. Dalakas M, Pezeshkpour G, Gravell M, Sever J. Polymyositis associated with AIDS retrovirus. *JAMA* 1986;256:2381-2383.
20. Nordstrom D, Petropolis A, Giorno R, Gates R, Reddy V. Inflammatory myopathy and acquired immunodeficiency syndrome. *Arth Rheum* 1989;32(4):475-479.
21. Scott J, Palmer E, Fischman A. HIV-associated myositis detected by radionuclide bone scanning. *J Nucl Med*: 1989; 30:556-558.
22. Wiley C, Nerenberg M, Cros D, Soto-Aguilar M. HTLV-I polymyositis in a patient also infected with the HIV virus. *NEJM* 1989;320:992-995.
23. Fleckenstein J, Burns D, Murphy F, Jayson H, Bonte F. Differential diagnosis of bacterial myositis in AIDS: evaluation with MR imaging. *Radiology* 1991;179:653-658.
24. Ledford D, Overman M, Gonzalvo A, Cali A, Mester S, Lockey R. Microsporidiosis myositis in a patient with the acquired immunodeficiency syndrome. *Ann Int Med* 1985;102(5):628-630.
25. Vartian C, Septimus E. Pyomyositis in an intravenous drug user with human immunodeficiency virus (letter). *Arch Int Med* 1988;148:2689.

26. Watts R, Hoffbrand B, Paton D, Davis J. Pyomyositis associated with human immunodeficiency virus infection. *Br Med J Clin Res* 1987;294:1524-1525.

27. Cornblath D. Treatment of the neuromuscular complications of human immunodeficiency virus infection. *Ann Neurol* 1988;23(Suppl):S88-91.

28. Cornblath D, McArthur J, Kennedy P, Witte A, Griffin J. Inflammatory demyelinating peripheral neuropathies associated with human T-cell lymphotropic virus type III infection. *Ann Neurol* 1987;21:32-40.

29. De LaMonte S, Gabuzda D, Ho D, Brown R, et al. Peripheral neuropathy in the acquired immunodeficiency syndrome. *Ann Neurol* 1988;23:485-492.

30. Eidelberg D, Sotrel A, Vogel A, et al. Progressive polyradiculopathy in acquired immune deficiency syndrome. *Neurology* 1986;36:912-916.

31. Grage M, Wiley C. Spinal cord and peripheral nerve pathology in AIDS: the roles of cytomegalovirus and human immunodeficiency virus. *Ann Neurol* 1989;25:561-566.

32. Parry G. Peripheral neuropathies associated with human immunodeficiency virus infection. *Ann Neurol* 1988;23(Suppl):S49-53.

33. Dalakas M, Pezeshkpour G, Flaherty M. Progressive nemaline (rod) myopathy associated with HIV infection (Letter). *NEJM* 1987;317:1602-1603.

34. Gonzalez M, Olney R, So Y, Greco C, McQuinn B, Miller R, deArmond S. Subacute structural myopathy associated with human immunodeficiency virus infection. *Arch Neurol* 1988;45:585-587.

35. Fleckenstein J, Haller R, Girson M, Peshock R. Focal muscle lesions in mitochondrial myopathy: MR imaging evaluation (Abst). *JRMI* 1992;2(Suppl):121.

36. Lamminen A. Magnetic resonance imaging of primary skeletal muscle diseases: patterns of distribution and severity of involvement. *Br J Radiol* 1990;63:946-950.

37. Whimbey E, Gold J, Polsky B, Dryjanski J, Hawkins C, Blevins A, Brannon P, Kiehn T, Brown A, Armstrong D. Bacteremia and fungemia in patients with the acquired immunodeficiency syndrome. *Ann Int Med* 1986;104:511-514.

38. Applegate G, Cohen A. Pyomyositis: early detection utilizing multiple imaging modalities. *Magn Reson Imag* 1991;9:187-193.

39. Fujino H, Kobayashi T, Goto I, Onitsuka H. Magnetic resonance imaging of the muscles in patients with polymyositis and dermatomyositis. *Muscle Nerve* 1991; 14:716-720.

40. Lamki L, Willis B. Radionuclide findings of pyomyositis. *Clin Nucl Med* 1982;10: 465-467.

41. Chiedozi L. Pyomyositis: a review of 205 cases in 112 patients. *Am J Surg* 1979;137: 255-259.

42. Bouvier J, Bocquet B, Lahneche B. Gallium-67 studies in a patient with multiple muscular abscesses. *Clin Nucl Med* 1986;11:807-808.

43. Datz F, Lewis S, Conrad M, Maravilla A, Parkey R. Pyomyositis diagnosed by radionuclide imaging and ultrasonography. *So Med J* 1980;73(5):649-651.

44. Howman-Giles R, McCauley D, Brown J. Multifocal pyomyositis diagnosis on technetium-99m MDP bone scan. *Clin Nucl Med* 1984;12:149-151.

45. Lachiewicz P, Hadler N. Spontaneous pyomyositis in a patient with Felty's syndrome: diagnosis using computerized CT. *So Med J* 1986;79:1047-1048.

46. Moore D, Delage G, Labelle H, Gauthier M. Peracute streptococcal pyomyositis: report of two cases and review of the literature. J *Ped Orthop* 1986;6:232-235.

47. Steinbach L, Tehranzadeh J, Fleckenstein J, Vanarthos W, Pais M. Musculoskeletal manifestations of human immunodeficiency virus (HIV) infection. *Radiology* 1993; 186:833-838.

48. Weinberg W, Dembert M. Tropical pyomyositis: delineation by gray-scale ultrasound. *Am J Trop Med* Hyg 1984;33(5):930-932.

49. Yuh W, Schreiber A, Montgomery W, Ehara S. Magnetic resonance imaging of pyomyositis. *Skeletal Radiol* 1988;17:190-193.

50. Drane W, Tipler B. Heterotopic ossification (myositis ossificans) in acquired immune deficiency syndrome. *Clin Nucl Med* 1987;12:433-434.

51. Tumeh S, Butler G, Maguire J, Nagel J. Pyogenic myositis: CT evaluation. *J Comput Assist Tomogr* 1988;12(6):1002-1005.

52. McLoughlin M. CT and percutaneous fine-needle aspiration biopsy in tropical myositis. *AJR* 1980;134:167-168.

53. Dalakas M, Gravell M, London W, Cunningham G, Sever J. Morphological changes of an inflammatory myopathy in Rhesus monkeys with simian acquired immunodeficiency syndrome. *Proc Soc Exp Biol Med* 1987;185:368-376.

54. Fleckenstein J, Watumull D, Conner K, Ezaki M, Greenlee R, Bryan W, Chason D, Parkey R, Peshock R, Purdy PD. Denervated human skeletal muscle: MR imaging evaluation. *Radiology* 1993;187:213-218.

55. Duewell S, Hagspiel K, Zuber J, von Schulthess G, Bollinger A, Fuchs W. Swollen lower extremity: role of MR imaging. *Radiology* 1992;184:227.

56. Musumeci R, Balzarini L, Ceglia E, et al. MRI in the evaluation of the swollen lower limb: a new diagnostic tool. In: Partsch H (ed), *Progress in Lymphology,* vol. 11. Amsterdam: Excerpta Medica 1988;387-390.

57. Hadjis N, Carr D, Banks L, Pflug J. The role of CT in the diagnosis of primary lymphedema of the lower limb. *AJR* 1985;144:361-364.

58. Wallgren-Pettersson, Kivisaari L, Jaaskelainen J, Lamminen A, Holberg C. Ultrasonography, CT and MRI of muscles in congenital nemaline myopathy. *Pediatr Neurol* 1990;6:20-28.

CHAPTER 5:

AIDS AND ARTHRITIS

Jamshid Tehranzadeh, M.D.
Michael Wenger, MD

INTRODUCTION

The association of AIDS and arthritis is well-documented in the literature, beginning with the first reports of Reiter's syndrome and psoriasis in HIV-infected persons in 1987 (1-3). Although these initial cases demonstrated patients with severe symptoms, it has now become clear that arthritis in HIV-infected persons has a wide spectrum of presentations ranging from mild arthralgias to very severe and disabling joint disorders. The presentation of arthritis may occur during any stage of the HIV disease (3-7). Winchester, et al(3) had a series of thirteen HIV-positive patients with arthritis. In his series, two patients had only immunologic abnormalities, six had AIDS-related complex, and five had classic manifestations of AIDS (8). In Berman's series (4), the majority of his patients had full-blown AIDS or an AIDS-associated infection; only one patient was asymptomatic. In Rowe's series (6), however, 11 of 36 (31%) patients were not known to be HIV-positive when they initially presented with arthritis. This has important implications since the possibility of AIDS must be suspected when any young adult presents with a seronegative arthritis (8).

Not only may arthritis be the first manifestation of AIDS, but some data suggests that the onset of arthritis in HIV-positive patients may actually lead to more rapid progression to AIDS (8) In the majority of patients the clinical course of arthritis is variable. Some patients develop a severe arthritis which does not respond well to treatment (3,6), while others have only short-lived joint symptoms which resolve without treatment. Still others present with acute synovitis which responds rapidly to anti-inflammatory medication. Arthritis has also been shown to recur (8).

The exact incidence of arthritis in HIV-positive patients is difficult to determine for several reasons. Many clinicians either overlook mild arthralgias or they do not associate arthritis with AIDS. Studies in Tampa, New York and Cleveland have reported the incidence of inflammatory arthritis in HIV-positive patients to be 16%(4) , 15%(9), and 25%(10), respectively. The prevalence for Reiter's syndrome was 10%(4), 4.6%(9), and 4.3%(10), respectively. A study from London, however, noted a minimum prevalence of inflammatory arthritis in approximately 1% of the HIV-infected population (7), while another study from San Francisco showed that the prevalence of arthritis in AIDS patients was 0.3% (11). It is likely that the true incidence of arthritis is underreported and clearly more detailed epidemiologic studies need to be performed.

The etiology of arthritis in AIDS patients is unclear. It is known that HIV binds to the membrane glycoprotein, CD4. The CD4 receptor is found predominantly on the T-helper lymphocytes. After binding to the CD4 receptor, the virus quickly enters the cell and kills the T-helper lymphocyte. Some researchers feel that the depletion of T-helper lymphocytes allow immune-regulated arthritides to occur. To further support this hypothesis, the peripheral blood CD4-positive lymphocyte counts have been found to be reduced in the majority of AIDS patients with arthritis (3,6,12). Others postulate that HIV may directly cause arthritis (13). HIV belongs to the subfamily of viruses called lentiviriniae (lentevirus). The best described lentevirus, visna virus, causes chronic arthritis in sheep (14). Another lentevirus, caprine arthritis-encephalitis virus (CAEV), also causes arthritis(14) and has been cultured from joint tissue. HIV has also been cultured from joint tissue(13), lending further strength to the argument that HIV may directly cause arthritis. The mere presence of HIV in joint fluid, however, may simply be a manifestation of widespread dissemination of the virus throughout the entire body, rather than implication of the virus for directly causing arthritis. Another cause of arthritis in AIDS patients may be infection from an enteric pathogen. Approximately one-third of all HIV-positive patients with Reiter's syndrome have a documented infection by an enteric pathogen (usually Shigella flexneri, Salmonella, Campylobacter jejeuni, Yersinia enterocolitica, and Yersinia pseudotuberculosis) (13). In another one third of patients, infections not traditionally linked to a reactive arthritis have been documented, most notably infection by mycobacterium avium intracellulare (15). Clearly, the pathogenetic mechanisms of AIDS and arthritis need to be further clarified. Perhaps one or a combination of all of these postulated mechanisms may play a role in the development of arthritis.

It is best to divide the arthritides in AIDS patients into five separate groups based on their different clinical presentations and their different responses to treatment. These five groups are: spondyloarthropathic arthritis (Reiter's syndrome, psoriatic arthritis, and undifferentiated spondyloarthropathy), HIV-associated arthritis, painful articular syndrome, acute symmetric polyarthritis, and septic arthritis (13). While it is convenient to separate these arthritides into groups, many patients defy precise classification and often present with overlapping features of several syndromes. Nevertheless, to gain better insight and understanding of the disease process, we will use this classification scheme throughout this chapter.

SPONDYLOARTHROPATHIC ARTHRITIS

Spondyloarthropathic arthritis consists of Reiter's syndrome, psoriatic arthritis, and undifferentiated spondyloarthropathy. They are the most common arthritides to affect AIDS patients. They are grouped together to emphasize the fact that they cannot be differentiated from each other based on their radiographic appearances. When patients have features of Reiter's syndrome or psoriatic arthritis but lack sufficient criteria to be classified into either category, they are given the diagnosis of undifferentiated spondyloarthropathy (13).

Reiter's syndrome was the first arthritis to be described in association with HIV infection (3). Since this time several articles have been published describing the association of HIV infection with Reiter's syndrome, psoriatic arthritis, and undifferentiated spondyloarthropathy (1,14-22). These arthritides have several similar radiographic and clinical features. The foot and ankle are the most commonly involved sites of inflammation. The most common finding in the foot is enthesopathy involving the Achilles tendon, plantar fascia, anterior and posterior tibial tendons, and the extensor tendons (13). The patient's enthesopathy can be so painful that it can cause confinement to a wheelchair. Some patients walk on the outer aspects of their feet, producing a wide-based gait known as "AIDS foot"(16). This wide-based gait can simulate the appearance of a peripheral neuropathy (13). Multidigit dactylitis also commonly occurs and may simulate the appearance of pedal edema. Osteolysis and pencil-in-cup deformities of the digits have been described. Knee inflammation is common, however, hip disease is rarely seen (20). In the upper extremities dactylitis is the typical radiographic finding. Wrist and elbow synovitis are uncommon. Enthesopathy is frequently seen in the upper extremities, usually presenting as lateral or medial epicondylitis, rotator cuff tendinitis, DeQuervain's disease, or flexor tendinitis (13).

One of the striking findings in AIDS patients with spondyloarthropathic arthritis is the lack of involvement of the axial skeleton. Some patients demonstrate sacroiliitis radiographically, however, no patient has had radiographic abnormalities in the spine. There appears to be no increased association of ankylosing spondylitis with HIV infection (23), which suggests that the pathogenic mechanisms that cause spondyloarthropathic arthritis in AIDS patients are different than the pathogenic mechanisms that cause ankylosing spondylitis. Although radiographic findings in the spine are typically absent in AIDS patients, some patients complain clinically of spinal pain and tenderness. In a series from London (6), 12 of 36 HIV-positive patients complained of spinal pain. Six patients had pain in the cervical region and 10 patients had pain in the thoracolumbar region, however, all of the patients had normal spine radiographs (8).

Skin and nail changes often accompany the spondyloarthropathic arthritides in AIDS patients. Although several forms of skin and nail disease have been described, seborrhea, psoriasis, and onychodystrophy are most commonly seen in this setting. Some reports have indicated that the presence of psoriasis and arthritis in HIV-positive patients imply a worse prognosis because these patients quickly develop severe immunodeficiency and opportunistic infections (13). Most patients with psoriasis develop an exacerbation of their skin disease when they develop AIDS (1,24-25). The psoriasis has also been reported to clear with end-stage AIDS (1). We encountered one HIV-positive patient who developed psoriatic arthritis of the hand and wrist as well as other joints following HIV conversion (Fig. 1).

Case History

A 26-year-old white male homosexual and IV drug abuser who was diagnosed with AIDS two years prior to admission has been admitted with *Pneumocystis carinii* pneumonia (PCP). He has had two other episodes of PCP on prior admissions. The past history is also significant for esophageal candidiasis, psoriatic arthritis, antral ulcer, disseminated mycobacterium avium intercellulare (MAI), history of elevated liver enzymes, and chronic anemia. On physical exam he is very cachectic and ill-appearing, and hypotensive. He has oral thrush, pale lips and conjunctiva, the skin is dry and scaly. Rectal exam reveals occult blood (OB) positive with grossly dark stool. The radiological examination showed multiple joint involvement in both hands and right wrist, both knees, and both ankles (Fig. 1). The patient was hydrated and transfused with blood and fresh frozen plasma and platelets. The blood pressure improved, however, active rectal bleeding necessitated several transfusions. He expired on the fifth hospitalization day.

Although psoriatic arthritis, Reiter's syndrome or undifferentiated spondyloarthropathy in HIV-positive patients cannot be clinically or radiographically distinguished from each other, there are some important features that are unique to AIDS patients with these arthritides. The arthritis and enthesopathies that occur in AIDS patients are often very severe and less responsive to anti-inflammatory drugs (23). Usually, psoriatic arthritis or Reiter's syndrome is a mild disease in patients without HIV infection and resolves slowly over 3 to 12 months (26). These arthritides in AIDS patients, however, are usually severe and often occur in association with immunodeficiency-related infections. Another important distinguishing feature of patients with HIV-associated

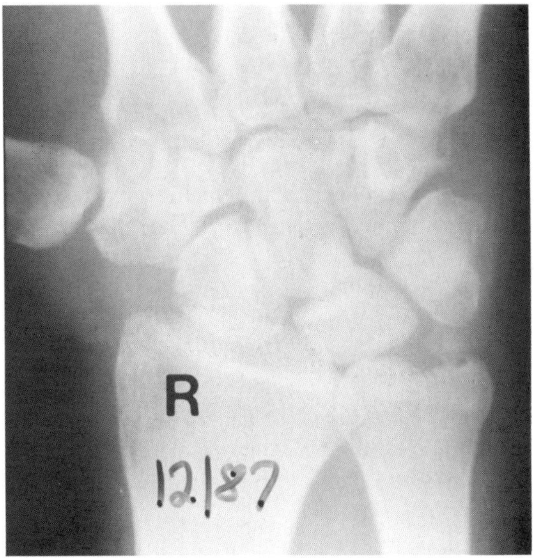

Figure 1-A

Psoriatic Arthritis. 27-year old man with AIDS who developed arthritis.
(A) AP and (B) lateral views of the right wrist shows soft tissue swelling around the wrist. Rotary subluxation of the scaphoid bone and ulnar translocation of carpal bones are noted.

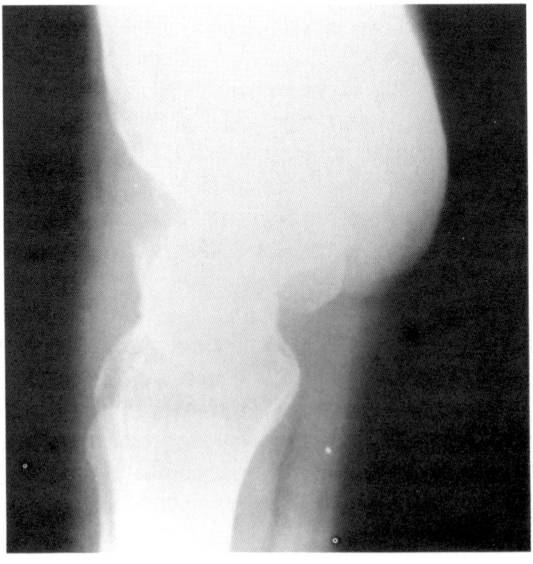

Figure 1-B

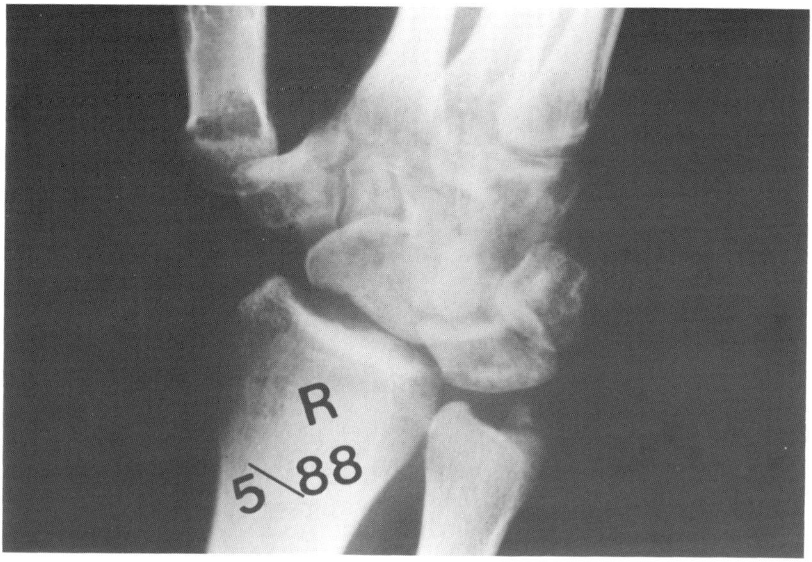

Figure 1-C
Oblique view of the right wrist six months later shows marked ulnar translocation of the carpal bones.

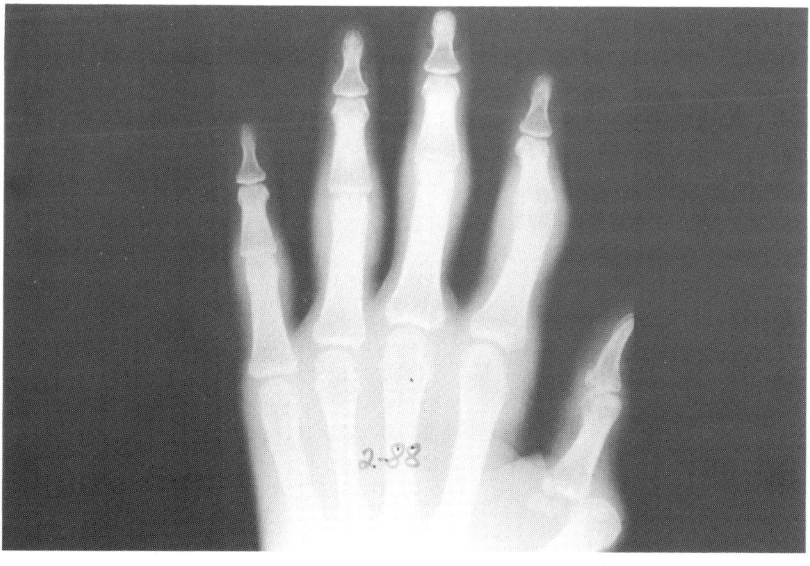

Figure 1-D
AP view of the left hand shows soft tissue swelling at the metacarpophalangeal and proximal interphalangeal joints and dislocation of the first metacarpophalangeal joint.

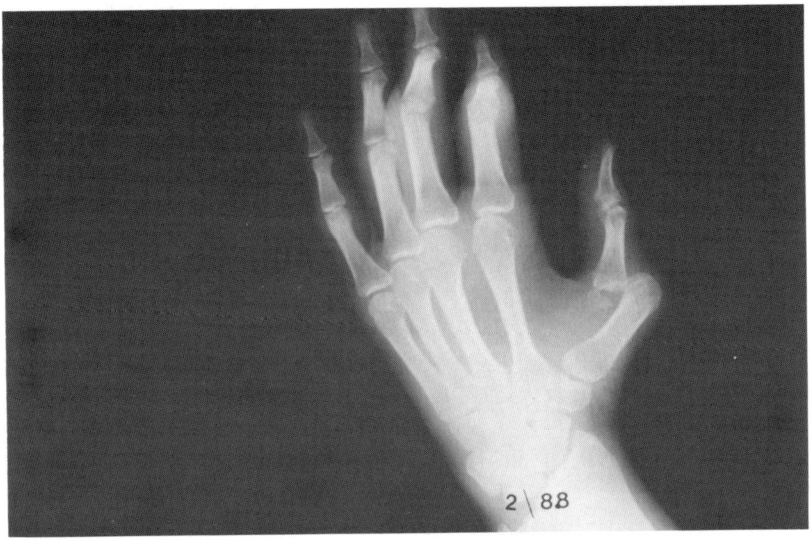

Figure 1-E

Oblique views of the left hand and wrist (I-E) shows marked increase in joint soft tissue swelling, dislocation of first metacarpophalangeal joint and Boutoniere deformities of the second, third and fourth fingers.

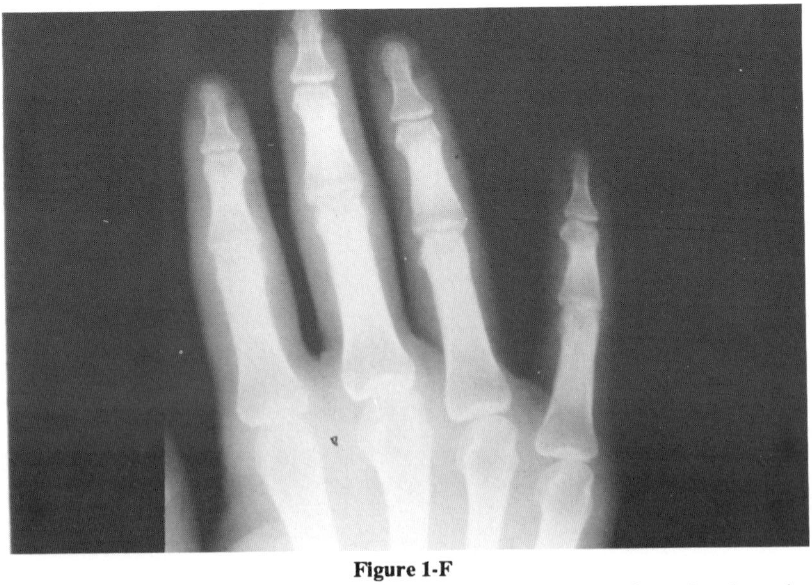

Figure 1-F

AP view of right hand shows soft tissue swelling of the metacarpophalangeal and proximal interphalangeal joints.

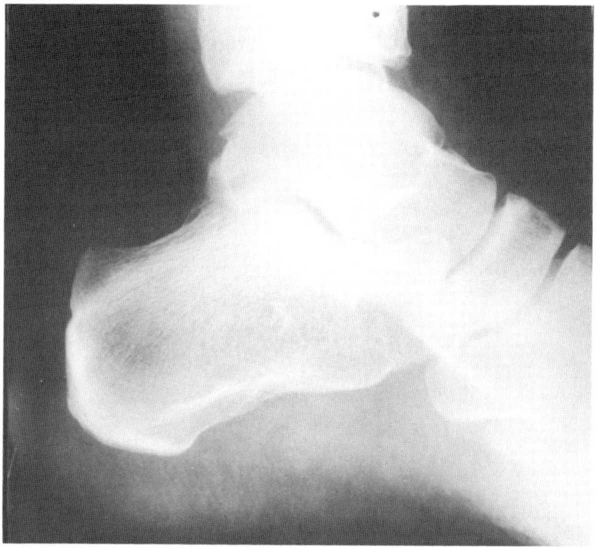

Figure 1-G
Lateral view of the left ankle shows soft tissue swelling around the joint.

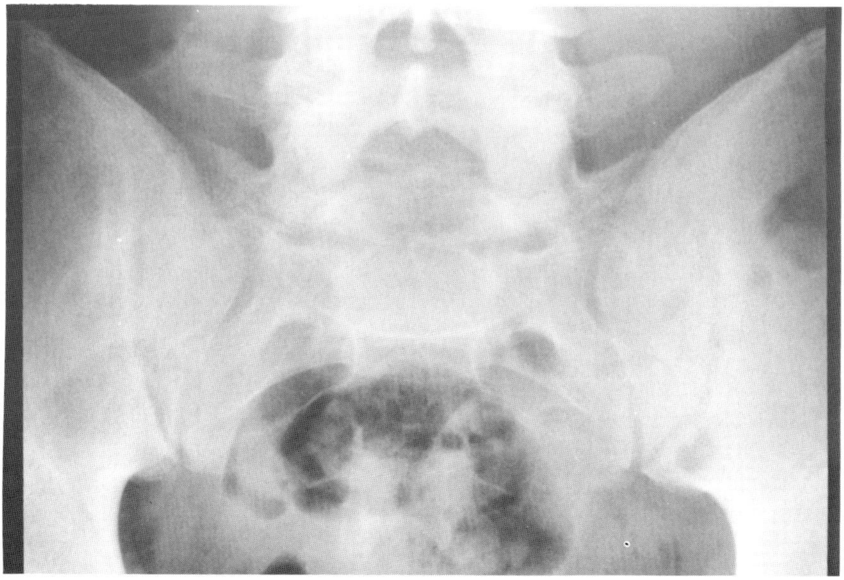

Figure 1-H
AP view of pelvis shows subtle cortical loss at both sacroiliac joints.

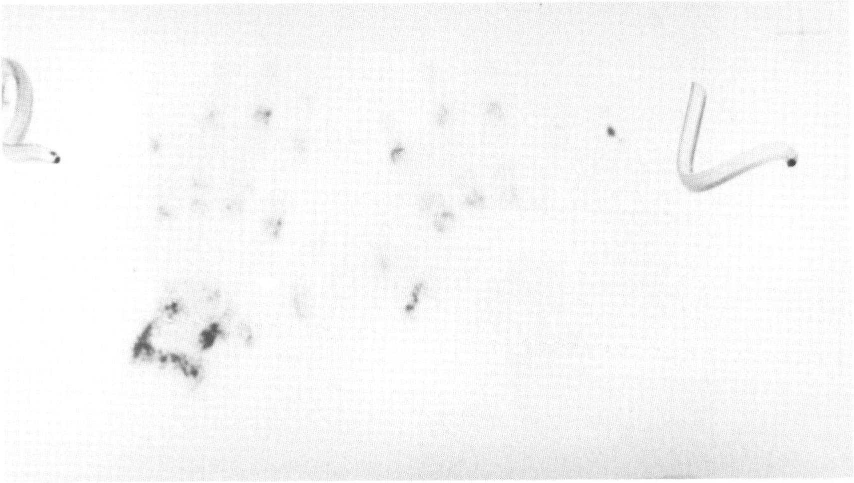

Figure 1-I
AP view of 99mTc-MDP bone scintigram shows multifoci of increased activity in the joints of both hands and right wrist indicating polyarthritis.

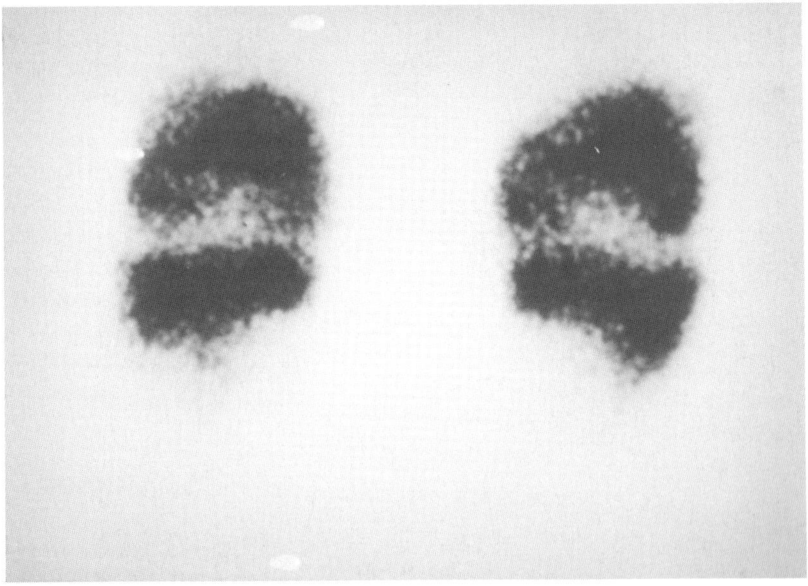

Figure 1-J
Posterior view of 99mTc-MDP bone scintigram shows diffuse increased activity in both knees.

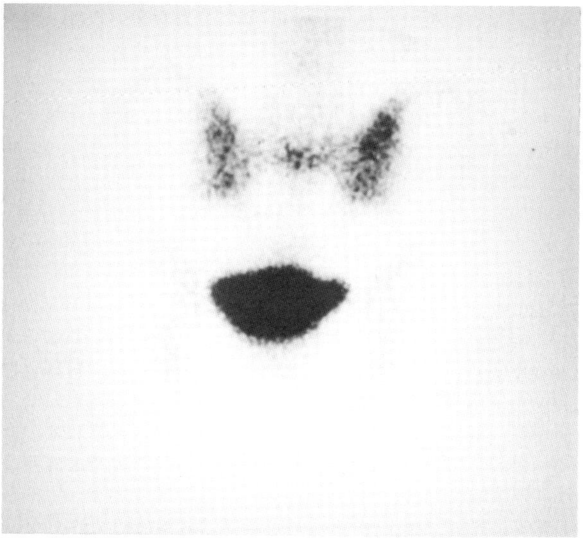

Figure 1-K
AP view of 99mTc-MDP bone scintigram shows only minimal increased activity at both sacro-iliac joints.

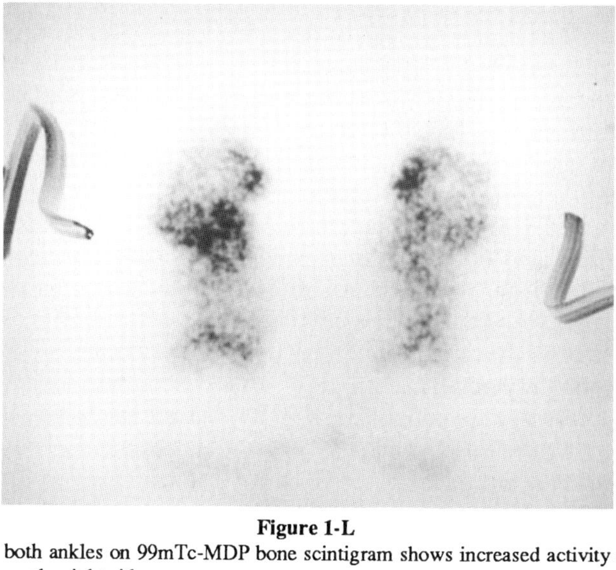

Figure 1-L
AP view of both ankles on 99mTc-MDP bone scintigram shows increased activity in both ankle joints, more on the right side.

spondyloarthropathies is striking muscle atrophy (13). The etiology for this muscular atrophy is unclear. Solomon, et al(13) speculate that the atrophy may be a result of neuropathy, myopathy, elevated levels of catabolic cytokines, or involuntary splinting of muscles. Physical therapy as well as appropriate splinting of inflamed tendons may help prevent the muscular atrophy (13).

The exact incidence of these spondyloarthropathic arthritides in HIV-positive patients and in the general population is controversial. The annual incidence of Reiter's syndrome in a non-HIV-infected population was estimated to be approximately 0.0035% (19), which was similar to a study by Noer(27), which reported 4 out of 100,000 military personnel with clinically documented Reiter's syndrome. Patients with HIV infection, however, have a 100-200-fold increased incidence of Reiter's syndrome. Two series (4,11) have reported the prevalence of Reiter's syndrome in the HIV-positive population to be in the range of 5%-10%. This data is conflicted in a study by Clark, et al(11) who reported a frequency of Reiter's syndrome in the male homosexual population to be 0.3% to 0.5%, however, there was no statistical difference between the incidence in HIV-positive and HIV-negative male homosexuals. Hochberg(28) also found no increased incidence of Reiter's syndrome in HIV-infected male homosexuals compared to male homosexuals without HIV infection. The studies by Clark and Hochberg may have been flawed since they relied on questionnaires to retrospectively analyze the data, and none of the patients in their studies were examined by rheumatologists. Despite the conflicting studies of Clark and Hochberg, current opinion appears to favor an increased incidence of Reiter's syndrome in the HIV-infected population.

There is also conflicting evidence to support the increased incidence of psoriatic arthritis in HIV-positive patients. The prevalence of psoriatic arthritis in the general population is approximately 0.01% to 0.14% (23). Winchester(22) and Berman(4) reported the incidence of psoriatic arthritis in the HIV-infected population to be 2% to 3%. Duvic(1), however, found no increased incidence of psoriatic arthritis in their HIV-positive patients. Obviously, much of the confusion arises from different criteria used to establish the diagnosis and different examiners. Future epidemiologic studies need to be performed to establish the exact incidence of the spondyloarthropathic arthritides in the HIV population. The etiology of the spondyloarthropathic arthritides in patients infected with HIV appears to be multifactorial. The HLA-B27 antigen appears to play a central role in the pathogenesis of Reiter's syndrome. Approximately 70% to 80% of non-HIV patients who possess the HLA-B27 antigen develop Reiter's syndrome, a frequency identical to that seen in HIV-positive patients with Reiter's syndrome (3,4,29). Moreover, it is well-known that HLA-B27 negative patients who develop reactive arthritis have a less severe arthritis and show fewer extra-articular manifestations of Reiter's syndrome (30). HLA-B27 is found in 6% to 10% of the normal population(23), therefore, the presence of the HLA-B27 antigen in an HIV-positive patient strongly indicates that he is likely to develop Reiter's syndrome. The HLA-B27 antigen, however, is not linked to the development of psoriatic arthritis or undifferentiated spondyloarthropathy (2-4,6,8).

Some authors(13) argue that Reiter's syndrome may be caused by infection. However, an enteric pathogen as a possible cause has only been detected in 33% of the cases. Nevertheless, an infectious etiology as a cause of Reiter's syndrome in some HIV-positive patients must be entertained.

It is tempting to speculate that a decrease in circulating CD4-positive lymphocytes may play a role in the development of spondyloarthropathic arthritides in HIV-positive patients. HIV attacks primarily the CD4-positive lymphocytes and several studies have shown that while the total white cell count is normal, the peripheral CD4-positive lymphocyte counts are reduced in the majority of HIV-positive patients with arthritis (3,6,12). It is possible that the depletion of CD4-positive lymphocytes may allow inciting organisms to proliferate or may alter the delicate balance of the immune system in some way to allow for the development of spondyloarthropathic arthritis.

It is interesting to note that while there is an increased incidence of spondyloarthropathic arthritis in the HIV population, there are some rheumatologic conditions that improve clinically when a patient is infected with HIV. Systemic lupus erythematosus (SLE) and rheumatoid arthritis (RA) have been reported to go into remission in patients with HIV infection (22). Tests for rheumatoid factor and antinuclear antibodies are routinely negative in HIV patients. It is unclear why SLE and RA should improve clinically with HIV infection, although it is easy to speculate that it may be the result of profound immunosuppression. There is a wide range of response to treatment in HIV-positive patients with spondyloarthropathic arthritis. Nonsteroidal anti-inflammatory drugs (NSAIDs) have been reported to cause moderate to good improvement in some patients (5). Others have reported little improvement with NSAIDs (3,6). Sulfasalazine and gold benefited two patients(3) but showed little effect on other patients (33). Intra-articular steroid injections have helped alleviate symptoms (4,6,7). Immunosuppressive agents and the use of Methotrexate are contraindicated because they may cause worsening of the immunodeficiency (3). More studies using antiviral agents, such as Zidovudine, need to be conducted. It is extremely important that septic arthritis is not mistaken clinically for spondyloarthropathic arthritis. Although they may appear clinically and radiographically similar, one must always perform synovial fluid cultures and institute broad-spectrum antibiotics if septic arthritis is suspected.

HIV-ASSOCIATED ARTHRITIS

HIV-associated arthritis was described by Rynes, et al(7) as a subacute, oligoarthritis typically affecting the knees and ankles. It was short in duration, usually lasting one to six weeks. The arthritis was often characterized by extreme pain. There was usually good response to nonsteroidal agents, rest, and intra-articular steroids (13).

The etiology of HIV-associated arthritis is unclear, however, many authors favor direct infection of the joint by HIV. Synovial biopsies have demonstrated only a mild cellular infiltrate, consisting mostly of mononuclear and plasma cells (7). Synovial fluid analysis typically reveals a noninflammatory reaction. HIV has been cultured from the synovial fluid (33). It is unlikely that this arthritis is related to the spondyloarthropathic arthritides because of the lack of enthesopathy, the short duration of symptoms, and the extreme pain and disability. None of the patients with HIV-associated arthritis have had a preceding infection and none have possessed the HLA-B27 antigen (13).

PAINFUL ARTICULAR SYNDROME

Berman(4) and Rynes(34) have described an arthralgia in HIV-positive patients consisting of extreme pain of very short duration, typically lasting 2 to 24 hours. The joint most commonly affected was the knee, however, the shoulder and elbow can also be involved. Patients usually responded well to NSAIDs. Some patients were confined to a wheelchair because of the extreme pain, the etiology of which is unknown. However, one must always consider HIV infection when examining a young patient with an intensely painful arthritis, especially involving the knee joint.

ACUTE SYMMETRIC POLYARTHRITIS

Rosenberg, et al(20) reported on four patients with symmetric polyarthritis involving the hands. Bentin and colleagues(35) described a similar case of a patient with symmetric polyarthritis. Although these patients had periarticular osteoporosis, marginal erosions, ulnar deviation, and swan-neck deformities consistent with rheumatoid arthritis, there were also several important distinctions. In Rosenberg's series the disease was acute in all of the patients, and in two patients there was marked new bone proliferation, highly unusual for rheumatoid arthritis. Most of the patients were male and the majority were rheumatoid factor negative. Benton's patient appeared to respond clinically to Azidothymidine (AZT). The cause of this arthritis is unclear, however, it does not appear to represent rheumatoid arthritis. As discussed previously, rheumatoid arthritis is rare in the HIV-positive population (31).

RHEUMATIC FEVER

Radcliffe argues that rheumatic fever ought to be listed along with other recognized causes of arthritis associated with HIV infection (36). Symptoms are related to delayed sensitivity immune reaction following group A streptococcal infection. Large joints of the extremities are typically affected in a migratory pattern, in conjunction with fever and often carditis. Roentgenographic findings are non-specific, revealing soft tissue swelling without evidence of osseous or cartilaginous destruction; there may be mild osteopenia. Both rheumatic fever and HIV cause CD4+ subset lymphopenia.

SEPTIC ARTHRITIS

It is surprising that septic arthritis is not very common in HIV-positive patients. It is important to always consider this diagnosis, because without proper treatment rapid joint destruction ensues. Septic arthritis can clinically simulate the typical reactive arthritis seen in AIDS patients. Synovial fluid culture is critical and, if infection is suspected, broad-spectrum antibiotics must be administered quickly. HIV patients are susceptible to the usual pathogens as well as opportunistic organisms. In intravenous drug abusers (IVDAs), the most common pathogen is bacterial, usually Staphylococcus aureus and Streptococcus pneumoniae(37) and there is a tendency to infect the axial joints. Opportunistic organisms most commonly infect non-IVDA patients. Infection may also spread to involve the bone or soft tissues. Rapid treatment is necessary to prevent further morbidity. Please also refer to the chapter on musculoskeletal infections in AIDS (Figs. 2, 3 & 4).

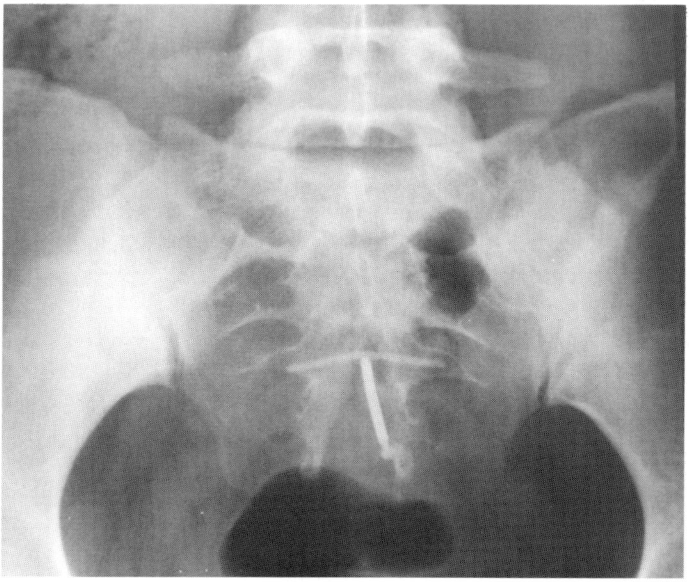

Figure 2

Sacroliitis. Young HIV-positive female with right sacroiliitis. AP view of the pelvis shows cortical indistinctness and sclerosis of the right sacroiliac joint.

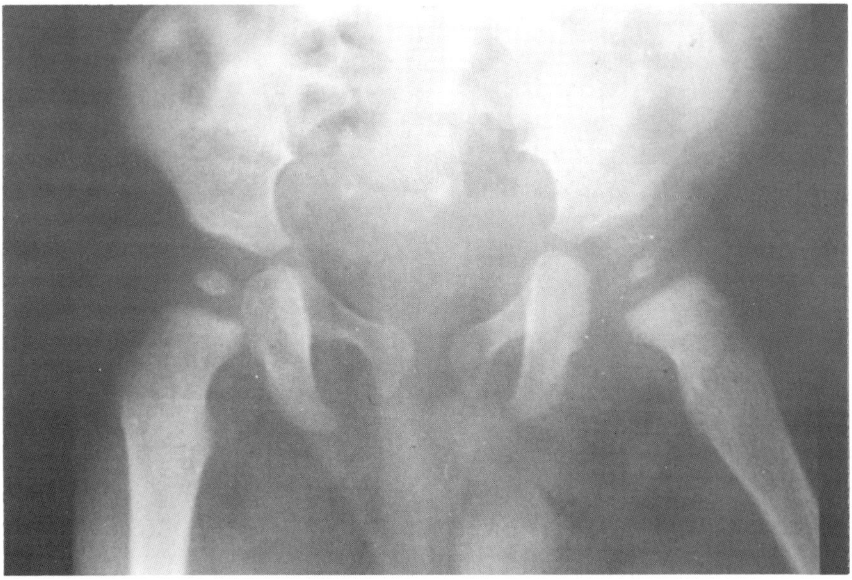

Figure 3.

Septic arthritis. HIV-positive child with left hip pain has acute septic arthritis of the left hip. AP view of the pelvis shows left hip joint widening due to effusion. Note cortical indistinctness of the femoral head and acetabulum.

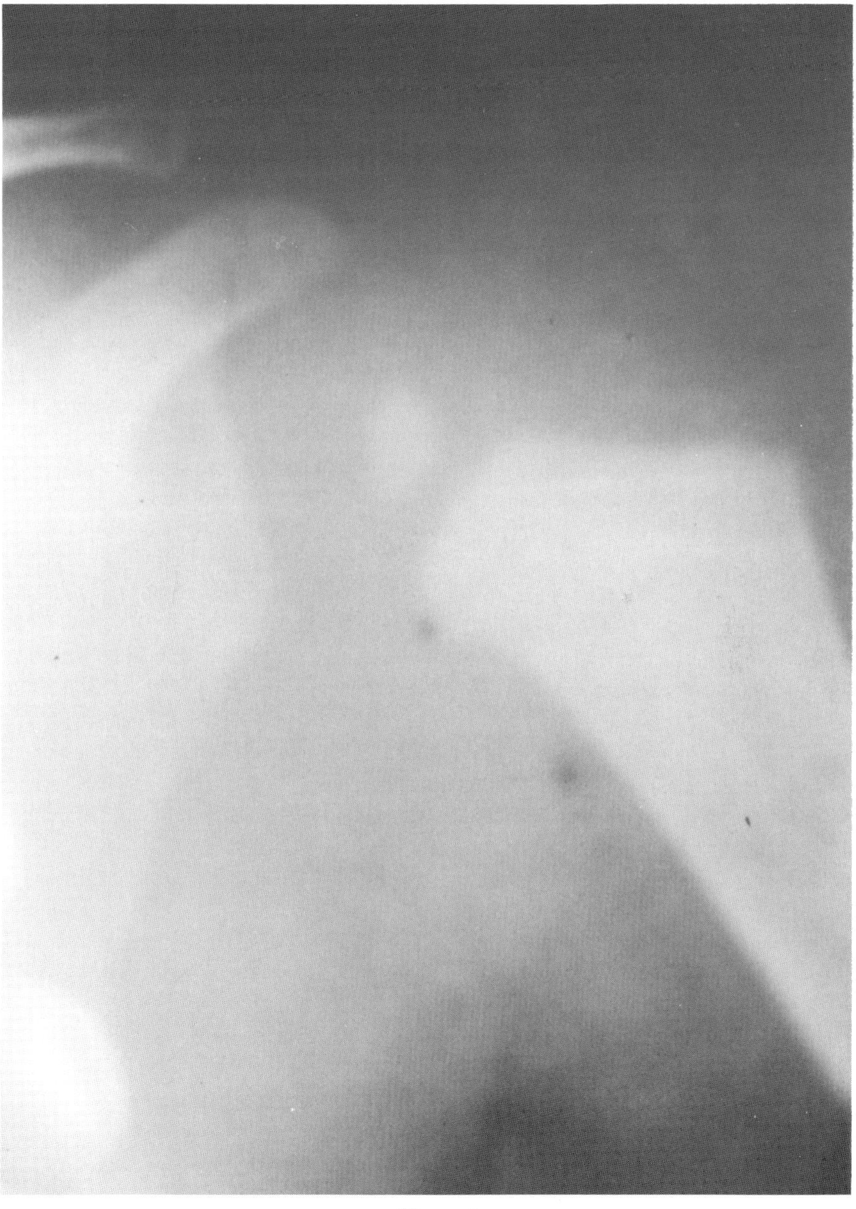

Figure 4

Septic arthritis. Septic arthritis of the left shoulder in an HIV-positive child. Note soft tissue swelling and widening of joint space.

CONCLUSION

Arthritis in AIDS patients can be conveniently classified into five groups: spondyloarthropathic arthritis, HIV-associated arthritis, painful articular syndrome, acute symmetric polyarthritis, and septic arthritis. While not all patients can be easily classified into one group, this classification scheme serves to separate these arthritides based on their different clinical features. Clinicians should be aware of how these arthritides present clinically and should always consider the diagnosis of HIV infection in a young patient presenting with a seronegative spondyloarthropathic arthritis.

REFERENCES

1. Duvic M, Johnson TM, Rapini RP, et al. Acquired immunodeficiency syndrome: associated psoriasis and Reiter's syndrome. *Arch Dermatol* 123:1622-1632,1987.
2. Oberlin F, Le Blonde V, Camus JP. Arthrites reactionnelles chez deux homosexuels a serologie HIV-positive. *La Presse Medicale* 16:355,1987.
3. Winchester R, Bernstein DH, Fischer HD, et al. The co-occurrence of Reiter's syndrome and acquired immunodeficiency. *Ann Int Med* 106:19-26,1987.
4. Berman A, Espinoza LR, Diaz JD, et al. Rheumatic manifestations of human immunodeficiency virus infection. *Am J Med* 85:59-64,1988.
5. Davies P, Stein M, Latif A, et al. Acute arthritis in Zimbabwean patients: possible relationship to human immunodeficiency virus infection. J *Rheumatol* 16:346-348, 1989.
6. Rowe IF, Forster SM, Seifert MH, et al. Rheumatological lesion in individuals with human immunodeficiency virus infection. *Q J Med* 73:1167-1184,1989.
7. Rynes RI, Goldenberg DL, DiGiacomo R, et al. Acquired immunodeficiency syndrome-associated arthritis. *Am J Med* 84:810-817,1988.
8. Keat A, Rowe I. Reiter's syndrome and associated arthritides. *Rheumatic Disease Clinics of North America* 17(1):25-33,1991.
9. Brancato L, Itescue S, Skovron M, et al. Aspects of the spectrum, prevalence and disease susceptibility determinants of Reiter's syndrome and related disorders associated with HIV infection. *Rheumatol Int* 9:137-141,1989.
10. Calabrese LH. The rheumatic manifestations of infection with human immunodeficiency virus. *Semin Arthritis Rheum* 18:225-239,1989.
11. Clark M, Kinsolving M, Chernhoff D. The prevalence of arthritis in two HIV-infected cohorts. *Arthritis Rheum* 32:S85, 1989.
12. Kaplan G, Ziza JM, Prier A, et al. Arthropathies inflammatories chez des malades infectes par le virus de immunodeficience humaine. *La Presse Medicale* 18:525-528, 1989.

13. Solomon G, Brancato L, Winchester R. An approach to the human immunodeficiency virus-positive patient with a spondyloarthropathic disease. *Rheumatic Disease Clinics of North America* 17(1):44-52,1991.
14. Narayan O, Cork LC. Lentiviral infections of sheep and goats: chronic pneumonia, leukoencephalomyelitis and arthritis. *Rev Infect Dis* 7:89-98,1985.
15. Winchester RW, Solomon G. Reiter's syndrome and acquired immunodeficiency. In: Espinoza L, Goldenberg D, Arnett F, et al (eds). *Infections in Rheumatic Diseases.* Orlando, Florida: Grune and Stratton, 343-347,1987.
16. Brancato LJ, Itescu S, Winchester RJ. Reiter's syndrome and related rheumatic conditions in HIV infection. *J Musculoskeletal Med* 15:32, August 1989.
17. Espinoza LR, Berman A, Vasey FB, et al. Psoriatic arthritis and acquired immunodeficiency syndrome. *Arthritis Rheum* 31:1034-1040,1988.
18. Forster SM, Seifert MH, Keat AC, et al. Inflammatory joint disease and human immunodeficiency virus infection. *Brit Med J* 296:1625-1627,1988.
19. Michet CJ, Machado EB, Ballard DJ, et al. Epidemiology of Reiter's syndrome in Rochester, Minnesota: 1950-1980. *Arthritis Rheum* 31:428-431,1988.
20. Rosenberg ZS, Norman A, Solomon G. Arthritis associated with HIV infection: radiographic manifestations. *Radiology* 173:171-176,1989.
21. Solomon G, Brancato LJ, Itescu S, et al. Arthritis, psoriasis, and related syndromes associated with HIV infection. (Abstract) *Arthritis Rheum* 31:512,1988.
22. Winchester RW, Brancato L, Itescu S, et al. Implications from the occurrence of Reiter's syndrome and related disorders in association with advanced HIV infection. *Scand J Rheum Suppl* 74:89-93,1988.
23. Arnett FC, Reveille JD, Duvic M. Psoriasis and psoriatic arthritis associated with human immunodeficiency virus infection. *Rheumatic Disease Clinics of North America* 17(1):59-78, 1991.
24. Johnson TM, Duvic M, Rapini RP, et al. AIDS exacerbates psoriasis. *NEJM* 313: 1415, 1985.
25. Kaplan MH, Sadick N, McNutt S, et al. Dermatologic findings and manifestations of acquired immunodeficiency syndrome (AIDS). *J Am Acad Dermatol* 16:485-506, 1987.
26. Arnett FC. Seronegative spondyloarthropathies. *Bull Rheum Dis* 37:1,1987.
27. Noer HR. An "experimental" epidemic of Reiter's syndrome. *JAMA* 198:693-698, 1966.
28. Hochberg MC, Fox R. HIV infection is not a risk factor for Reiter's syndrome. (Abstract) *Clin Res* 37:318A, 1990.
29. Reveille JD, Conant MA, Duvic M. HIV-associated psoriasis, psoriatic arthritis and Reiter's syndrome: a disease continuum? *Arthritis Rheum* 33(10):1574-1578,1990.
30. Monteagudo I, Rivera J, Lopez-Longo J, et al. AIDS and rheumatic manifestations in patients addicted to drugs. An analysis of 106 cases. *J Rheumatol* 18(7): 1040, 1991.

31. Furie RA. Effects of human immunodeficiency virus infection on the expression of rheumatic illness. *Rheumatic Disease Clinics of North America* 17(1):177-187,1991.
32. Espinoza LR, Aguilar JL, Berman A, et al. Rheumatic manifestations associated with human immunodeficiency virus infection. *Arthritis Rheum* 32(12):1615-1622, 1989.
33. Withrington RH, Cornes P, Harris JRW, et al. Isolation of human immunodeficiency virus from synovial fluid of a patient with reactive arthritis. *Brit Med J* 294:484, 1987.
34. Rynes RI. Painful rheumatic syndromes associated with human immunodeficiency virus infection. *Rheumatic Disease Clinics of North America* 17(1):83,1991.
35. Bentin J, Feremans W, Pasteels J, et al. Chronic acquired immunodeficiency syndrome-associated arthritis: a synovial ultrastructural study. *Arthritis Rheum* 33(2):268-273, 1990.
36. Radcliffe KW, McLean KA, Benbow AG. Acute rheumatic fever in human immunodeficiency virus infection. J *Infect* 1991 Mar;22(2):187-189.
37. Goldenberg DL. Septic arthritis and other infections of rheumatologic significance. *Rheumatic Disease Clinics of North America* 17(1):149-156,1991.

CHAPTER 6:

MUSCULOSKELETAL LYMPHOMA IN AIDS

Jamshid Tehranzadeh, M.D.
Debra Butler, M.D.

Lymphoma is a malignant tumor of lymphoid tissue which is categorized into two groups — Hodgkin's disease (distinguished by characteristic clinical features and morphologic features such as Reed-Sternberg giant cells) and non-Hodgkin's lymphoma (NHL) (1). We will focus our discussion to AIDS-related lymphoma (ARL), which is primarily of the non-Hodgkin's type. Non-Hodgkin's lymphoma has been reported at a much higher frequency in AIDS patients since 1982 (with an incidence approximately 60 times that of the general population). Non-Hodgkin's lymphoma meets one of the criteria for the diagnosis of AIDS in patients infected with the human immunodeficiency virus (HIV) (2,3). Hodgkin's lymphoma has not been definitively reported with a greater frequency in patients with AIDS, and it remains controversial whether it is a manifestation of AIDS in an HIV-infected patient.

In the non-AIDS population, NHL develops in both intranodal lymphoid tissue (65% of cases) and extranodal lymphoid tissue of parenchymal organs (35% of cases) (1). Sites of extranodal involvement include the gastrointestinal system, oropharynx, central nervous system (CNS), bone marrow, pulmonary system, liver, skin, and testes. NHL includes a wide spectrum of disorders and is classified into different types. Historically, three main classification systems exist: the Rappaport classification and the newer, widely accepted Working Formulation, which are both based on morphologic features; and the Lukes-Collins classification based on immunologic and cytochemical features.

Lymphoma (both NHL and Hodgkin's disease) has unusual features in AIDS patients. At the time of presentation in AIDS patients, the disease tends to be more advanced (stage III or IV), more commonly extranodal and more aggressive. It also has a worse prognosis (4-7). In addition, the majority of AIDS patients with NHL have high-grade B-cell types with small non-cleaved or large immunoblastic types (8). Ziegler et al reviewed 90 patients with ARL and demonstrated a marked increase in extranodal involvement, including the CNS, bone marrow, abdominal organs, and mucocutaneous sites (7).

Musculoskeletal lymphoma is not common in patients with AIDS. We will include a brief discussion of the more common sites of involvement such as the gastrointestinal tract, central nervous system, and chest. Involvement of the gastrointestinal tract may resemble Kaposi sarcoma with multiple nodular masses or diffuse bulky tumors (9). Isolated masses in the gastrointestinal tract without additional lesions elsewhere are less common (2). Focal masses may involve the stomach, small bowel or colon. Involvement of the stomach usually appears as infiltrating lesions, ulcers, masses, or thickened rugal folds. Lesions often mimic the appearance of carcinoma (10).

Other abdominal manifestations of lymphoma in AIDS patients include involvement of the liver, spleen, omentum, kidneys, abdominal and pelvic lymph nodes, and the retroperitoneum (2). Lymphomatous involvement of the liver is much more common in AIDS patients than in non-AIDS patients and may present as diffuse hepatomegaly without focal lesions apparent on CT, or may vary from single to multiple hypodense lesions. A similar, less common situation may occur in the spleen presenting with multiple hypodense lesions on CT (2).

Gross infiltration of the psoas muscle mimicking infection and gross infiltration of the omentum can occur (peritoneal lymphomatosis) (2). A focal or infiltrative mass may uncommonly be seen in the kidney. Diffuse lymphomatous involvement of retroperitoneal and mesenteric nodes may also occur. However, adenopathy is nonspecific and can also be seen in AIDS patients with reactive lymphoid hyperplasia, mycobacterial infection, and Kaposi sarcoma (2,11). Abdominal adenopathy with nodes of greater than 1.5 cm in diameter is usually not related to reactive hyperplasia and is most commonly seen in NHL, *Mycobacterium avium intracellulare*, or Kaposi sarcoma (11). Lymphomatous involvement of the myocardium has also been described with the presence of intracardiac masses and pericardial effusion (2,4,12).

AIDS-related Lymphoma of the Central Nervous System

Central nervous system (CNS) lymphoma in both AIDS and non-AIDS patients can be primary or secondary. There is a greater prevalence of both primary and secondary CNS lymphoma in the AIDS population, as compared to the non-AIDS population (13). Primary CNS lymphoma is a rare disease in the pediatric population, mainly seen in patients with immunodeficiency disorders or with immunosuppressed states (such as transplant patients) and is now being seen with greater frequency secondary to AIDS (14,15). The EBV is thought to play a role in the etiology of CNS lymphoma in the pediatric AIDS population (16).

The CT appearances of primary and secondary CNS lymphoma are identical (17). CT typically demonstrates single or multiple focal homogeneous lesions, which are hyper- or iso-intense with the brain parenchyma and may have a surrounding area of low attenuation edema (13-15, 18). There is usually peripheral ring enhancement or total homogeneous enhancement of the lesion after administration of IV contrast. Other nonspecific findings include nodular or confluent areas of periventricular enhancement or corpus callosum involvement (19). Magnetic resonance (MR) may be more sensitive but, again, is nonspecific as are the CT findings, and biopsy is often required for diagnosis.

Baumgartner et al studied 55 patients with AIDS and pathologically proven CNS lymphoma; 37% of patients had unifocal mass lesions and 63% had multifocal mass lesions on post-contrast CT scans (20). Pathologic findings were also interesting in that 18 of the 55 cases were of the small-cell, noncleaved type and 17 of the 55 were of the large-cell, immunoblastic type.

AIDS-related Lymphoma of the Chest

Lymphomatous involvement of the chest is a relatively rare manifestation of AIDS compared to the more frequent pulmonary manifestations, such as infection with *Pneumocystis carinii pneumonia* (PCP), *Mycobacterium tuberculosis,* and *Mycobacterium avium intracellulare* (21). The radiographic appearance of ARL involving the chest is variable and includes pleural effusion, interstitial and alveolar disease, pulmonary nodules, and mediastinal adenopathy (5,12,22). In a study by Sider et al, the majority of patients presented with multiple sites of thoracic involvement, with the two most frequent manifestations being pleural effusion and lung disease (12). The presence of thoracic lymphadenopathy is significant because it is not a feature of PCP infection or of persistent generalized lymphadenopathy, but can be seen in chronic infection, including fungal or tuberculous (23). ^{67}Ga scanning may show focal uptake by the involved lymph nodes.

Musculoskeletal Lymphoma in AIDS

Primary musculoskeletal lymphoma is a rare disease but can involve bone, muscle, skin, and subcutaneous tissues (24). Primary NHL of the bone represents only 4% of bone tumors (25), however, secondary involvement of the bone in patients with both Hodgkin's and NHL is common, especially in children (24). The most common site of bone involvement in primary NHL is the lower extremities. Although primary bone involvement is rare in Hodgkin's lymphoma, metastatic involvement of the bone is common (24).

There have been very few reported cases in the literature of lymphoma of the musculoskeletal system in AIDS patients (4,25,26). Banerjee et al present a 42-year-old HIV-positive male with a lytic lesion in the right femoral neck and on the anterior surface of L5 with bony destruction and an adjacent soft tissue mass (4). Biopsy of the femur demonstrated bone marrow involvement. The second patient presented by Banerjee was a 65-year-old HIV-positive male with pathologic fracture of the distal left femur, in which biopsy revealed an immunoblastic high-grade NHL. Langford et al reported five cases of primary malignant B-cell lymphoma involving either the maxilla or mandible (26).

NHL of bone in the general population usually presents as a permeative osteolytic lesion with cortical destruction (24,27,28). The tumor may also be sclerotic and mixed and may have a long, indistinct transition zone. Periosteal reaction and an associated soft tissue mass may be present, and there may be extensive extraosseous and bone marrow involvement. Pathologic fracture may be one of the presenting features. CT and MR are the modalities of choice for imaging the bone and soft tissue changes and both are complementary studies.

The usual differential diagnosis for musculoskeletal lymphoma in the non-AIDS population, depending upon age and clinical presentation, includes osteosarcoma, Ewing's tumor, metastatic disease, and chronic osteomyelitis or myositis (24). The differential diagnosis of a lytic bone lesion in the AIDS population may differ slightly and includes lymphoma, a recently described AIDS syndrome of bacillary angiomatosis (thought to be caused by a bacterium similar to the bacillus isolated in cat scratch disease), and Kaposi's sarcoma (29). It should be kept in mind, however, that lytic lesions of bone are not very common in AIDS patients.

Lymphoma involving the skeletal muscle is also rare, especially the primary type (30). Involvement of the muscle can occur by metastatic spread, direct extension from adjacent bone or lymph node, or most uncommonly as a primary lesion (31). Decreased attenuation as compared to normal muscle tissue on CT and slight enhancement on post-contrast CT have also been described (30,32).

In the series reported by Steinbach et al (33), seven men had biopsy-proven involvement of the musculoskeletal system with non-Hodgkin's lymphoma. Conventional radiographs and CT scans were obtained in all of these patients. In four of these patients, lymphoma was first diagnosed in the skeletal system without known extraskeletal sites. Patients included a 42-year-old man with a retrobulbar mass invading the medial wall of the orbit and destroying the ethmoid and maxillary sinuses (Fig. 1); a 29-year-old man with lytic destruction of the left shoulder joint, including the scapula (Fig. 2); a 40-year-old man with sclerotic lesions in the pelvis secondary to lymphoma (Fig. 3); a 36-year-old man with lytic involvement of the skull, right hip and ischium; and a 39-year-old man with a previous diagnosis of lymphoma who developed lymphomatous lytic lesions in multiple vertebral bodies and in the pelvis (Fig. 4). Two men, aged 36 and 61 years, respectively, had lymphomatous involvement of thigh musculature with known involvement elsewhere, which was well demonstrated on MR images.

CT, bone scan and MRI are the main imaging modalities for evaluating musculoskeletal lymphoma. MR may better define the extent of soft tissue (Figs. 5 & 6) and bone marrow involvement, but it is nonspecific and biopsy is necessary for diagnosis (Figs. 7 & 8).

HIV-Associated Hodgkin's Disease

There is no definite evidence of an absolute increase in the number of Hodgkin's disease cases in the AIDS population. However, an increased incidence of Hodgkin's disease among high-risk groups, such as intravenous drug abusers in New York prisons and homosexuals in New Orleans, has been noted. The large number of cases of AIDS-associated Hodgkin's disease reported to date clearly indicates a more aggressive course for the disease and an alteration of the clinical features in the setting of AIDS. Of 109 patients with Hodgkin's disease, 84% presented with Stage III or Stage IV disease, compared with the expected rate of only 40% in a non-HIV-infected population. Despite the high response to conventional therapy, patients with HIV-associated Hodgkin's disease have a high mortality rate due to opportunistic infections (34).

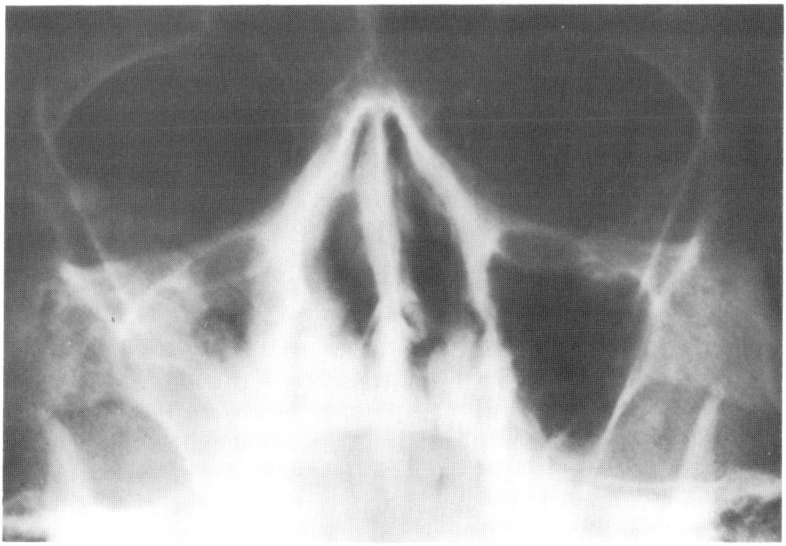

Figure 1-A

Lymphoma of Orbit. Lymphoma of the right orbit extending to the right maxillary sinus and nasal cavity. (Courtesy of Sharon E. Meagher, Miami, Florida). Water's view shows opacification of the left maxillary sinus.

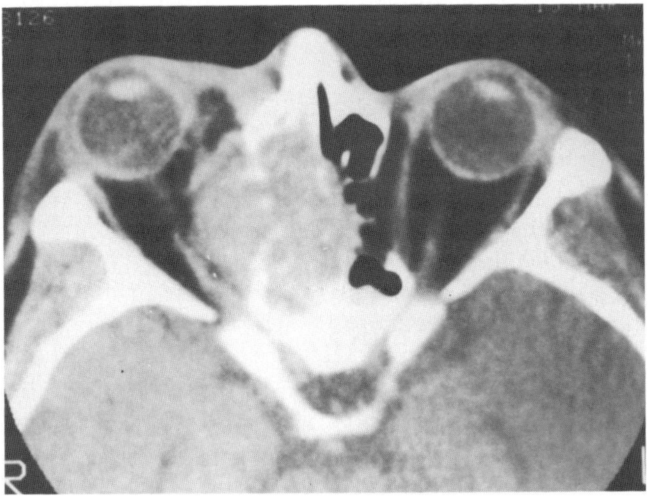

Figure 1-B

CT scan shows retrobulbar mass extending into the left maxillary, ethmoid sinuses and left nasal cavity.

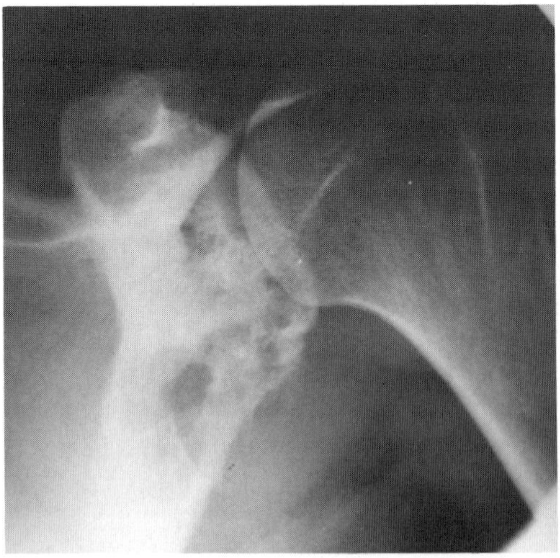

Figure 2-A

Lymphoma of Scapula. Lymphoma of scapula in an AIDS patient. (From Steinbach, et al: Radiology 1993;186:833-838, with permission) This is a 29-year-old white Caucasian male (guitar player) with left shoulder pain. AP plain radiograph of the left shoulder shows marked lytic and destructive changes of the glenoid process extending to the body of the scapula with aggressive periosteal reaction and large soft tissue mass.

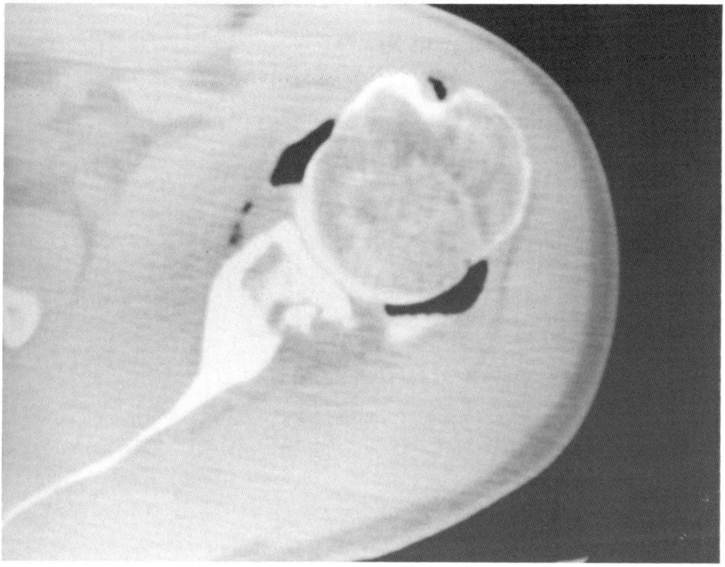

Figure 2-B

CT following shoulder arthrogram shows lytic changes of the glenoid process with anterior and posterior soft tissue mass. The articular cartilage remains intact.

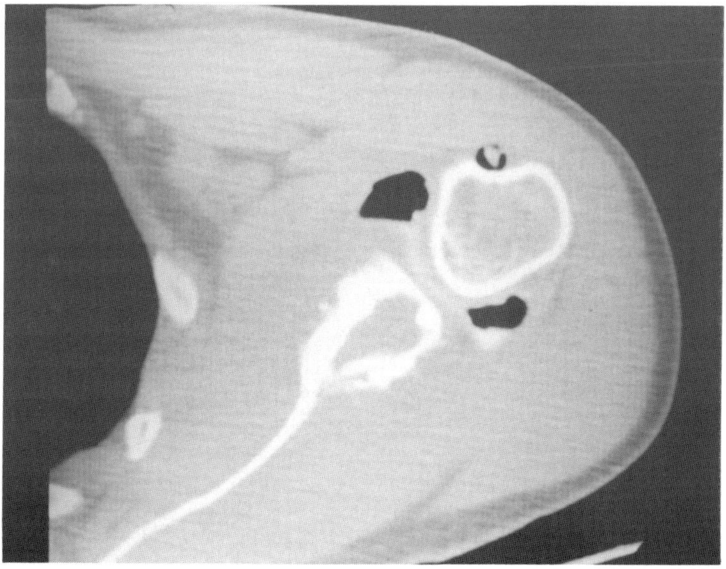

Figure 2-C

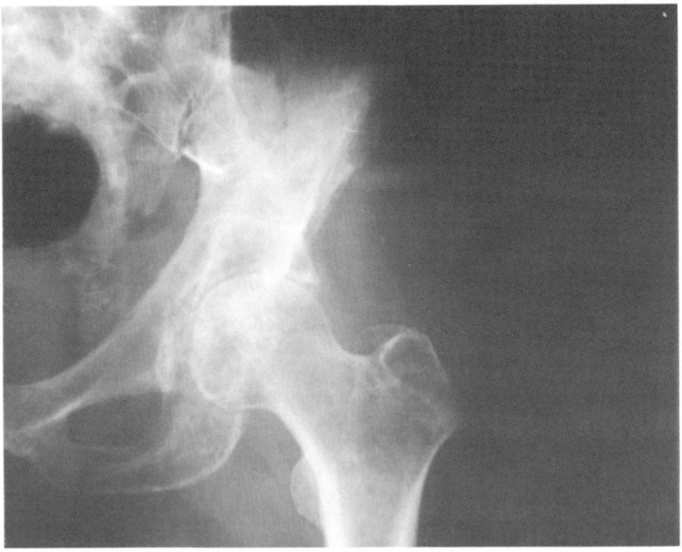

Figure 3-A

Lymphoma of Pelvis. Lymphoma of the pelvis in an AIDS patient. This is a 40-year-old homosexual man with pain in the left hemipelvis. A & B. Original radiographs (A) and two-month follow-up (B) radiograph of the left hemipelvis show marked lytic and sclerotic changes of the left inominate bone. Note pathologic fracture of ischium (arrow).

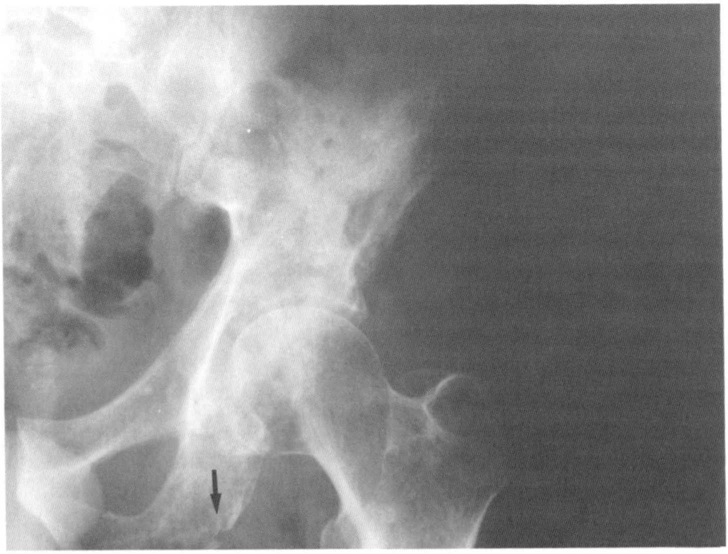

Figure 3-B

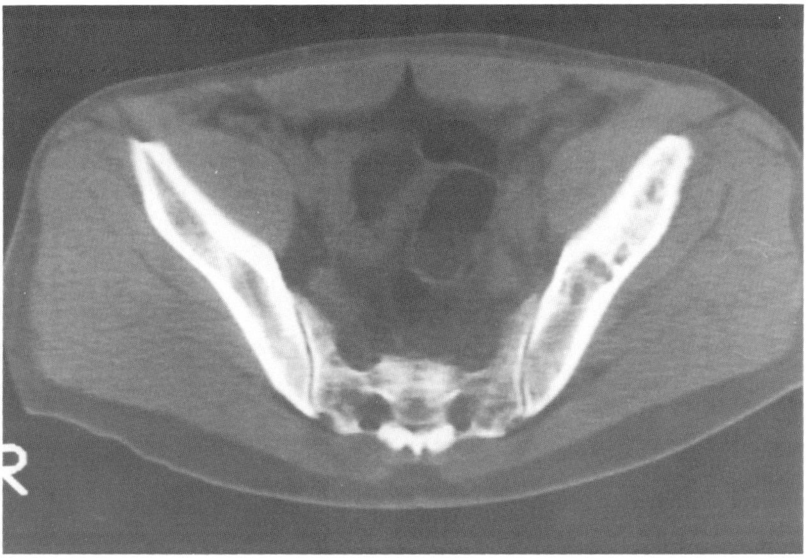

Figure 3-C

Original CT (C) and two-month follow-up CT of the pelvis (D& E) show mixed lytic and sclerotic lesions of the pelvis with internal and external pelvic soft tissue mass on the left side.

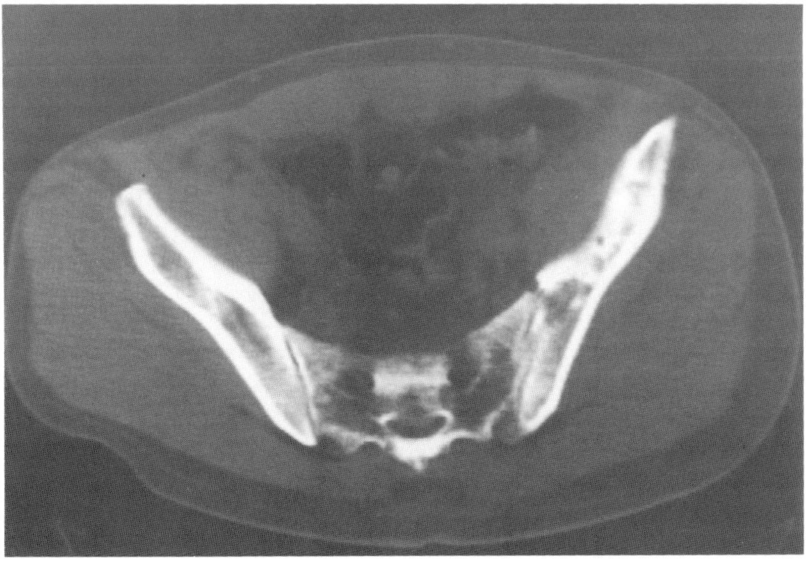

Figure 3-D

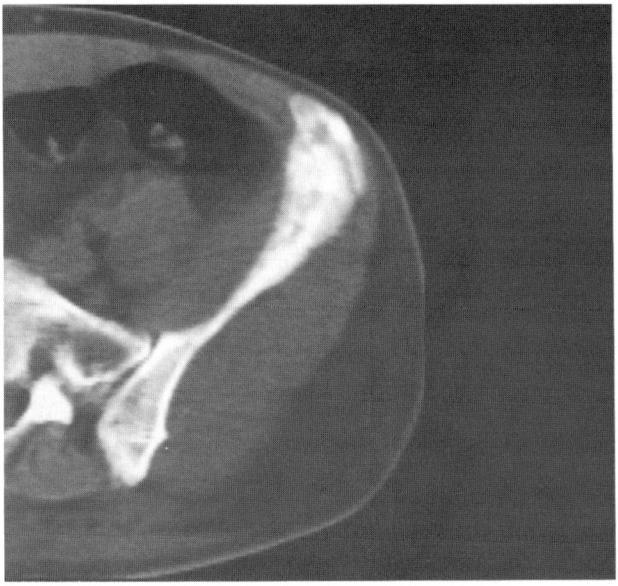

Figure 3-E

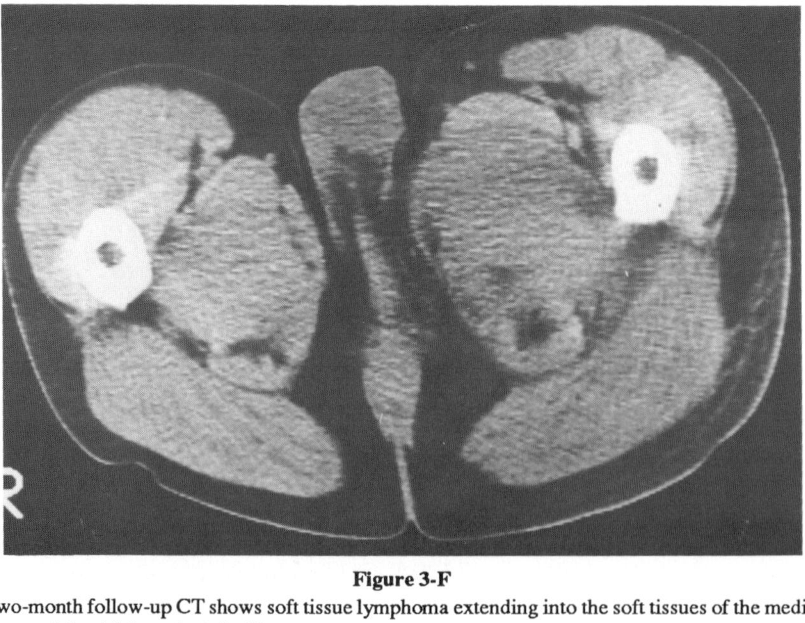

Figure 3-F

Two-month follow-up CT shows soft tissue lymphoma extending into the soft tissues of the medial aspect of the thigh on the left side.

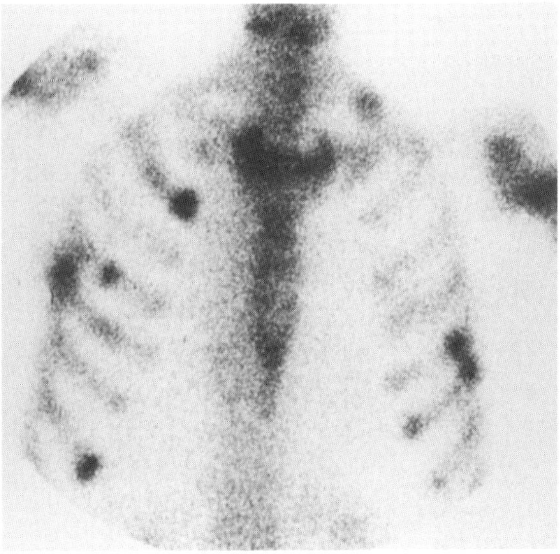

Figure 4-A

Multiple Skeletal Lymphomas. Multiple skeletal lymphomas in an AIDS patient. This is a 39-year-old man with AIDS and multiple bone pain. Multiple areas of focal increased uptake throughout the thoracic rib cage and both proximal humeri are noted.

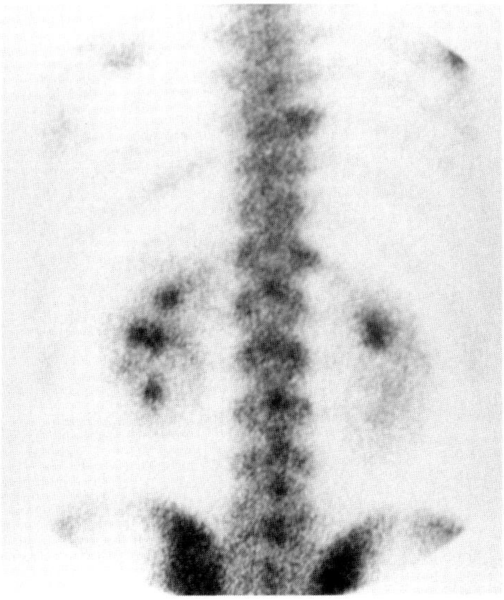

Figure 4-B

Focal areas of increased activity in the spine were also seen.

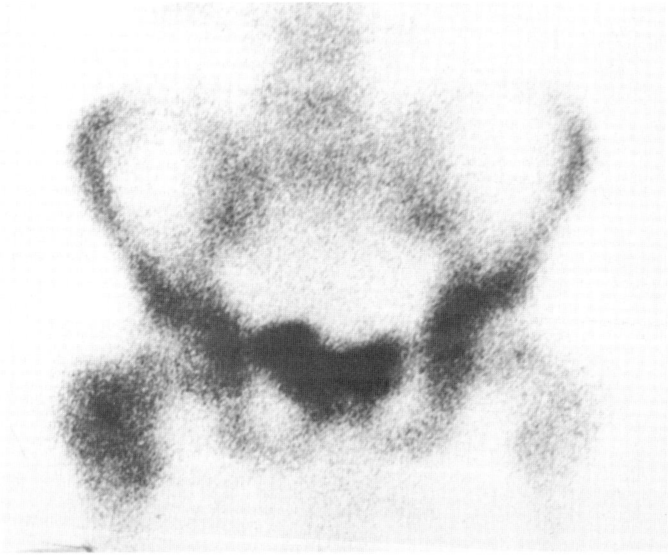

Figure 4-C
There is diffuse increased activity in the pelvis and right proximal femur.

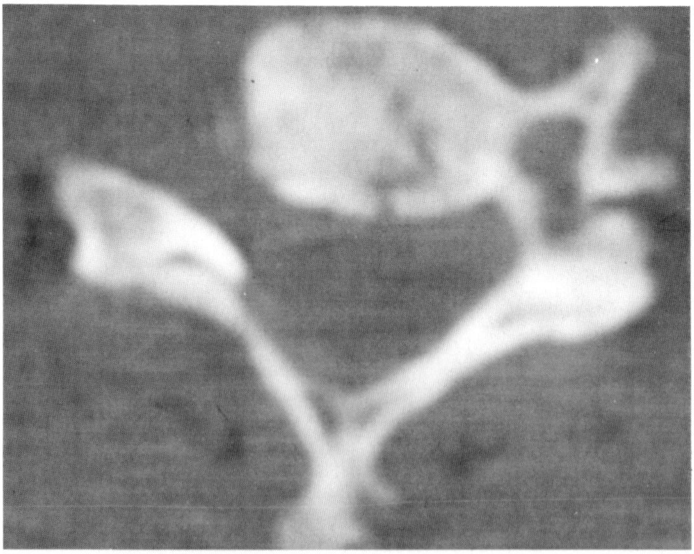

Figure 4-D
Lytic and sclerotic changes of the vertebral body of the cervical spine with pathologic fracture are noted.

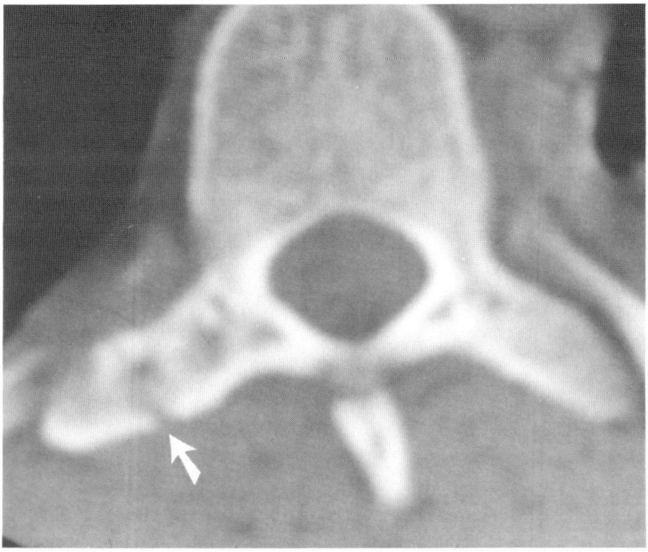

Figure 4-E

Lytic changes with pathologic fracture (arrow) of the transverse process of the thoracic spine on the right side with adjacent soft tissue mass are noted.

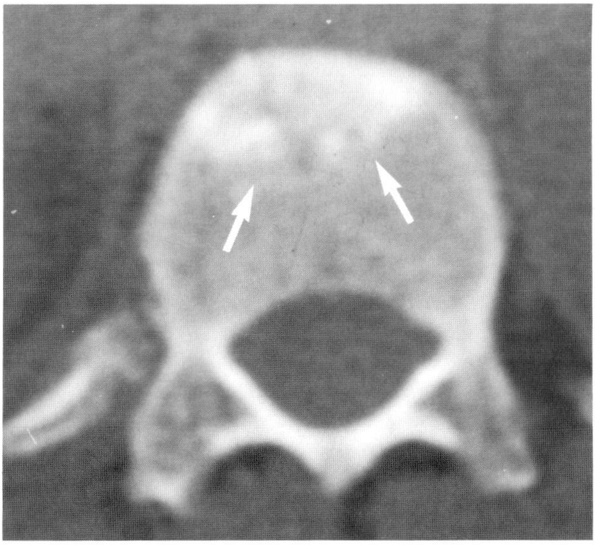

Figure 4-F

Sclerotic involvement of the thoracic vertebrae, indicating osteoblastic lesion in the anterior vertebral body (arrows).

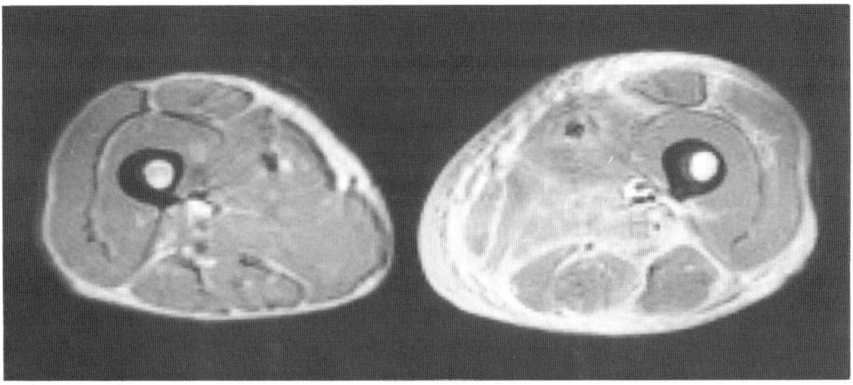

Figure 5-A

Lymphoma. This is a 61-year-old HIV-positive male diagnosed with intravascular large-cell cutaneous lymphoma. He had ascites, pleural fluid and developed a swollen leg. (Courtesy of John Barr, M.D.) Axial proton density MR image (TR/TE 2100/34) of the thigh shows lymphomatous infiltration in the posterior muscles of the left thigh.

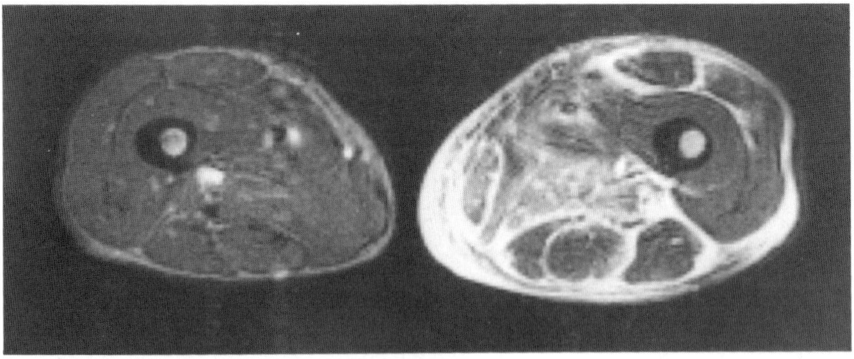

Figure 5-B

Axial T2-weighted images (TR/TE 2100/80) obtained at the same level show lymphomatous infiltration at the same region.

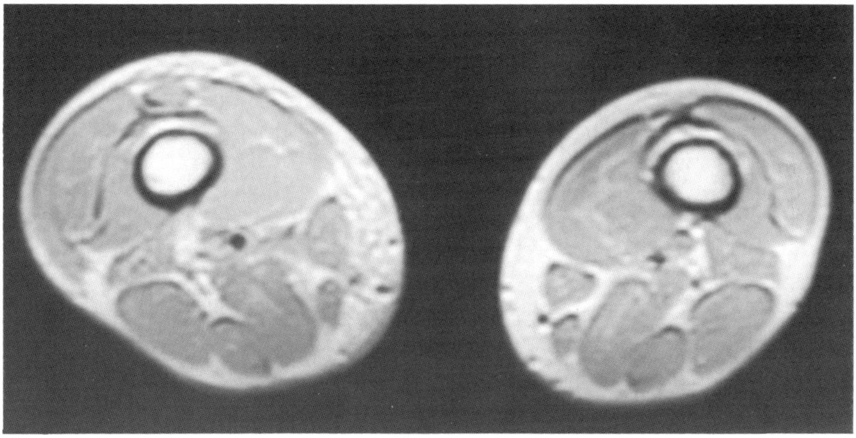

Figure 6-A

Poorly differentiated lymphoma. This is a 40-year-old HIV-positive male with poorly differentiated lymphoma. He presented with a one-month history of low back pain and right thigh swelling. (Courtesy of Lynne Steinbach, M.D.) Axial PDWI (TR/TE 2500/12) of the thigh. It is difficult to appreciate any abnormality in the musculature on this proton density image.

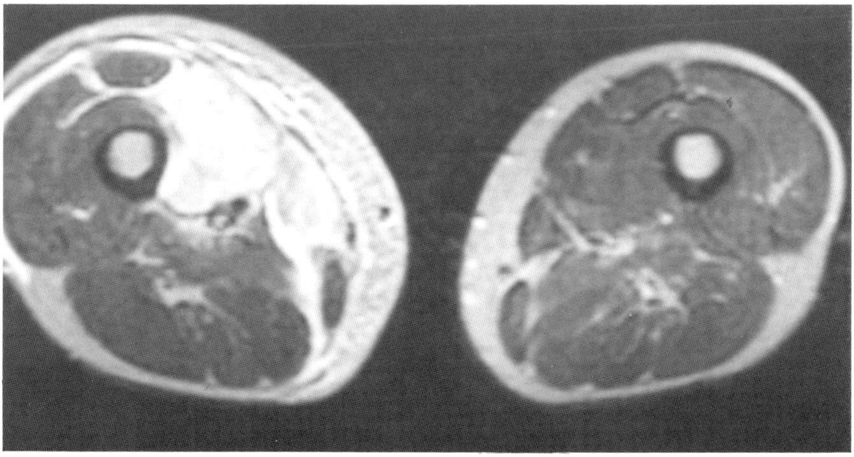

Figure 6-B

Axial T2WI (TR/TE 2500/80) demonstrates high signal intensity indicating infiltration of sartorius and vastus medialis muscles in the right thigh. This lesion enhanced with Gadolinium (not shown).

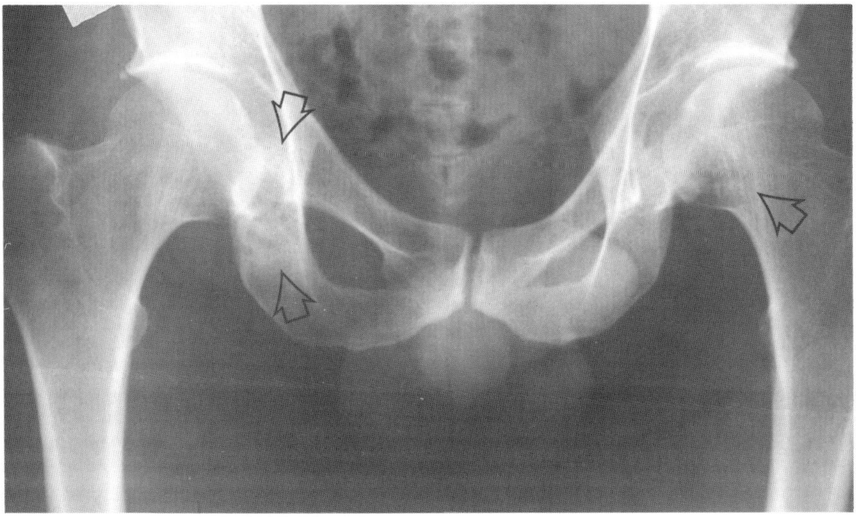

Figure 7

Multifocal Skeletal Lymphoma. This is a 35-year-old HIV-positive male with multifocal skeletal high-grade non-Hodgkin's lymphoma. The lymphoma was previously treated with radiation and chemotherapy. Skeletal involvement included multifocal lesions of the pelvis including ischium and ilium, proximal femur, ribs, and calvarium. Biopsy was taken from one of the ribs. Patient also had axillary and retroperitoneal lymphadenopathy and lymphomatous involvement of the liver. He also had a prior history of Kaposi sarcoma, hemophilus influenza pneumonia, and CMV retinitis. AP radiograph of the lower pelvis shows mixed area of sclerosis and lucency involving the right ischium and focal lucency of proximal left femur (arrows), consistent with metastatic lymphoma.

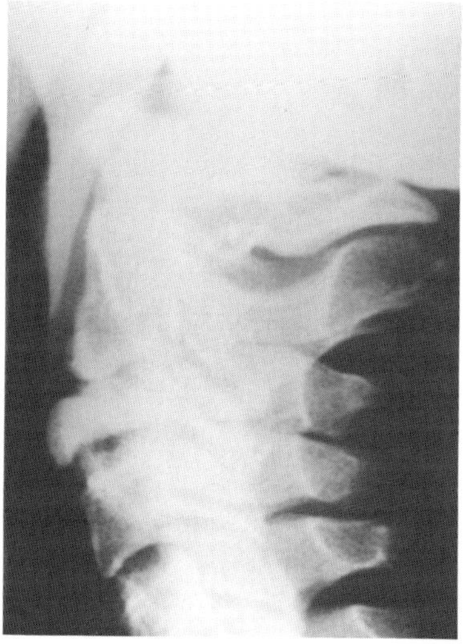

Figure 8-A

Multifocal Skeletal Lymphoma. 32-year-old HIV-positive man with history of neck pain and back pain, has multifocal lymphoma of the cervical (C3) and thoracic (T3) spine. (Courtesy of Roger Kerr, Los Angeles, California). Lateral AP radiograph of the cervical spine shows flattening and sclerosis of C3 cervical vertebra.

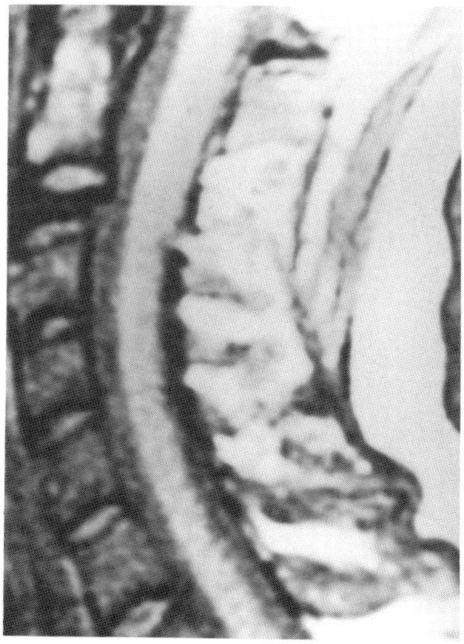

Figure 8-B

Sagittal T1-weighted image (TR 600/TE 26) without Gadolinium demonstrates collapse of the C3 vertebral body. The bone is decreased in signal intensity.

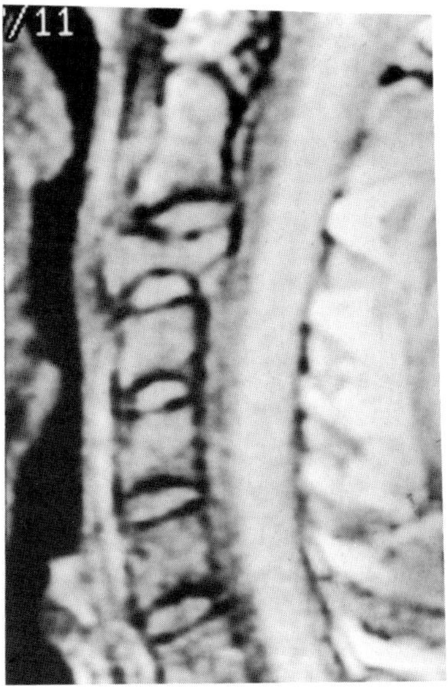

Figure 8-C
Sagittal T1-weighted image with gadolilium demonstrates enhancement of C3.

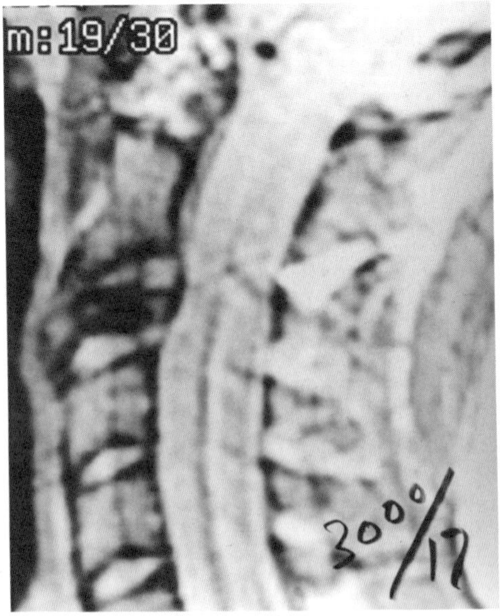

Figure 8-D
Sagittal proton-density weighted image (TR 3000/TE 17) of the collapsed C3 vertebral body.

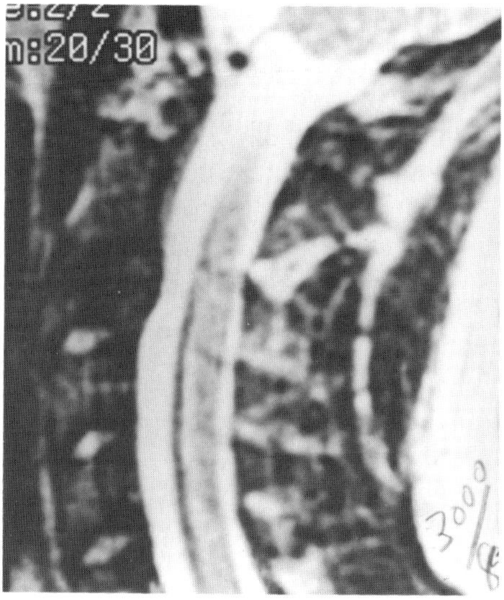

Figure 8-E
T2-weighted image (3000/85) shows collapse of C3 with low signal intensity.

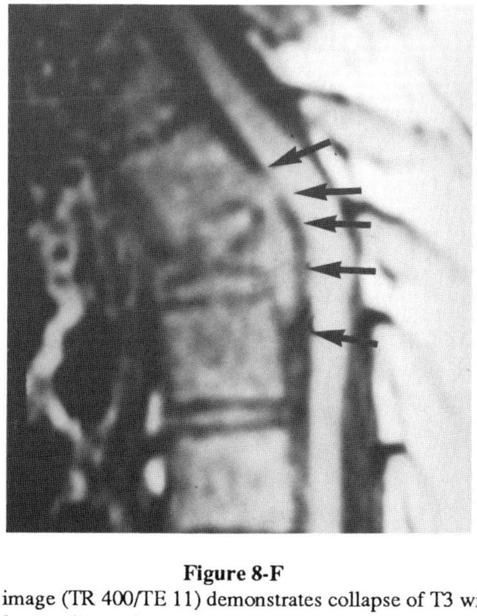

Figure 8-F
Sagittal T1-weighted image (TR 400/TE 11) demonstrates collapse of T3 with a soft tissue mass at the anterior epidupal space (arrows).

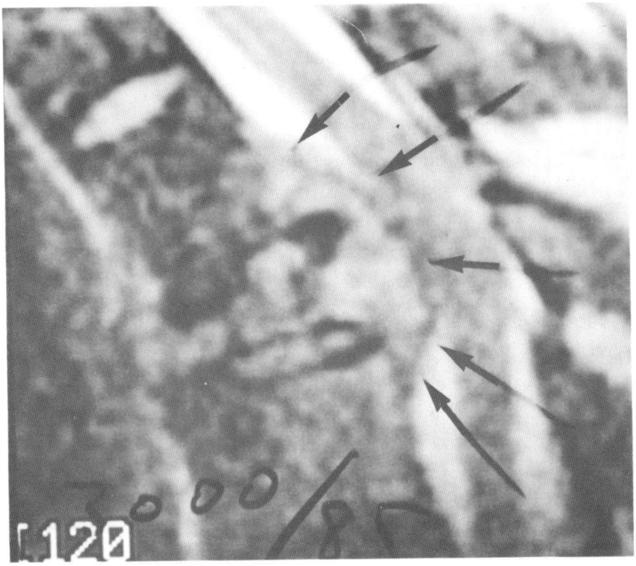

Figure 8-G

T2-weighted image (TR 3000/TE 85) of upper thoracic spine shows collapse of T3 with soft tissue mass at anterior epidural space (arrows).

REFERENCES

1. Coltan RS, Kumar V, Robbins SL. Robbins Pathologic Basis of Disease, 4th ed. W.B. Saunders Co., 1989, pp 708-716.
2. Townsend RR. CT of AIDS-related lymphoma. *Am J Roentgenol* 1991 May;156(5): 969-974.
3. Beral V, Peterman T, Berkelman R, Jaffe H. AIDS-associated non-Hodgkin's lymphoma. *Lancet* 1991;337:805-809.
4. Banerjee AK, Marshall T, Gazzard BG. The radiological appearance of bone lymphoma in AIDS. *Clin Radiol* 1992 Mar;45(3):169-171.
5. Naidich DP, McGuinness G. Pulmonary manifestations of AIDS. CT and radiographic correlations. *Rad Clin North Am* 1991 Sep;29(5):999-1017.
6. Nyberg DA, Federle MP. AIDS-related Kaposi sarcoma and lymphomas. *Semin Radiol* 1987 Jan;22(1):54-65.
7. Ziegler JL, Beckstead JA, Volberding PA, et al. Non-Hodgkin's lymphoma in 90 homosexual men. Relation to generalized lymphadenopathy and the acquired immune deficiency syndrome. *NEJM* 1984;311:565-570.
8. Kaplan LD, Abrams DI, Feigal E, McGrath M, Kahn J, Naville P, et al. AIDS associated non-Hodgkin's lymphoma in San Francisco. *JAMA* 1989;261:719-724.

9. Wall SD. Gastrointestinal imaging in AIDS - luminal gastrointestinal tract. *Gastroenterol Clin North Am* 1988 Sep;17(3):523-533.
10. Falcone S, Murphy BJ, Weinfeld A. Gastric manifestations of AIDS: radiographic findings on upper gastrointestinal examination. *Gastrointest Radiol* 1991 Spring; 16(2):95-98.
11. Jeffrey RB, Nyberg DA, Bottles K, Abrams DI, Federle MP, Wall SD, et al. Abdominal CT in acquired immunodeficiency syndrome. *AJR* 1986 Jan;146:7-13.
12. Sider L, Weiss AJ, Smith MD, vonRoenn JH, Glassroth J. Varied appearance of AIDS-related lymphoma in the chest. *Radiology* 1989 Jun;171(3):629-632.
13. Levy MR, Bredesen DE, Rosenblum ML. Neurological manifestations of the acquired immunodeficiency syndrome (AIDS). Experience at UCSF and review of the literature. J *Neurosurg* 1985 Apr;62:475-95.
14. Epstein LG, Frederick JD, Joshi VV, Connor EM, Oleske JM, Kay D, et al. Primary lymphoma of the central nervous system in children with acquired immunodeficiency syndrome. *Pediatrics* 1988 Sep;82(3):355-363.
15. Goldstein J, Dickson DW, Rubenstein A, Woods W, Mincer F, Belman AL, Davis L. Primary central nervous system lymphoma in a pediatric patient with acquired immune deficiency syndrome. Treatment with radiation therapy. *Cancer* 1990 Dec; 66(12):2503-2508.
16. Andiman WA, Martin K, Rubinstein A, Pahwa S, Eastman R, Katz B, et al. Opportunistic lymphoproliferations associated with Epstein-Barr viral DNA in infants and children with AIDS. *Lancet* 1985 Dec;28:1390-1393.
17. Weingarten K, Zimmerman RD. CT of intracranial lymphoma. *Semin Ultras CT MR* 1986 Mar;7(1):9-17.
18. Goldstein JD, Zeifer B, Choa C, Moser FG, Dickson DW, Hirschfeld AD, Davis L. CT appearance of primary CNS lymphoma in patients with acquired immunodeficiency syndrome. *J Comput Assist Tomogr* 1991;15(1):39-44.
19. Ramsey RG, Geremia GK. CNS complication of AIDS: CT & MR findings. *AJR* 1988 Sep;151:449-454.
20. Baumgartner JE, Rachlin JR, Beckstead JH, Meeker TC, Levy RM, Wara WM, et al. Primary central nervous system lymphomas: natural history and response to radiation therapy in 55 patients with acquired immunodeficiency syndrome. *J Neurosurg* 1990 Aug;73:206-211.
21. Poulton TB. Chest manifestations of AIDS. *Amer Fam Phys* 1992 Jan;45:163-168.
22. Polish LB, Cohn DL, Ryder JW, Myers M, O'Brien RF. Pulmonary non-Hodgkin's lymphoma in AIDS. *Chest* 1989 Dec;96(6):1321-1326.
23. Stern RG, Gamsu G, Golden JA, Hirji M, Webb WR, Abrams DI. Intrathoracic adenopathy: differential feature of AIDS and diffuse lymphadenopathy syndrome. *AJR* 1984 Apr;142:689-692.
24. Malloy PC, Fishman EK, Magid D. Lymphoma of bone, muscle and skin. CT findings. *AJR* 1992 Oct;159:805-809.

25. Sabbaoh M, Meyer O, DeBandt M, Salomon-Ceron D, Perronne C, Rosenbaum W, Tremoliere F, Kahn MF. Bone manifestations associated with acquired immunodeficiency syndrome (AIDS). *Annales de Medicine Interne* 1992;143(1):50-56.
26. Langford A, Dienemann D, Schurman D, Pohle HD, Pauli G, Stein H, Reichart P. Oral manifestations of AIDS-associated non-Hodgkin's lymphoma. *Int J Oral Maxilofac Surg* 1991 Jun;20(3):136-141.
27. Rosenberg SA, Diamond HD, Jaslowitz B, Craver CF. Lymphosarcoma: review of 1,269 cases. *Medicine* 1961;40:31-84.
28. Coppes MJ, Patte C, Couanet D, Caillaud JM, Salloum E, Brugieres L, et al.Childhood malignant lymphoma of bone. *Med Pediatr Oncol* 1991;19(1):22-27.
29. Baron AL, Steinbach LS, LeBoit PE, Mills CM, Gee JH, Berger TG. Osteolytic lesions and bacillary angiomatosis in HIV infection: radiologic differentiation from AIDS-related Kaposi sarcoma. *Radiology* 1990;177: 77-81
30. Grunshaw ND, Chalmers AG. Skeletal muscle lymphoma. *Clin Radiol* 1992;45:399-400.
31. Kandel RA, Bedard YC, Pritzker KPH, Luk SC. Lymphoma presenting as an intramuscular small cell malignant tumor. *Cancer* 1984;53:1586-1589.
32. Scally J, Garrett A. Primary extranodal lymphoma in muscle. *Brit J Radiol* 1989; 62(733):81.
33. Steinbach LS, Tehranzadeh J, Fleckenstein JL, Vanarthos WJ, Pais MJ. Human immunodeficiency virus infection: musculoskeletal manifestations. *Radiology* 1993;186:833-838.
34. Safai B, Diaz B, Schwartz J. Malignant neoplasms associated with human immunodeficiency virus infection. *CA - A Cancer Journal for Clinicians* March/April 1992;42(2):74-95.

CHAPTER 7:

KAPOSI SARCOMA: SKELETAL MANIFESTATIONS

Lynne S. Steinbach, M.D.

BACKGROUND

Patients infected with the human immunodeficiency virus (HIV) have an increased likelihood of developing certain malignancies. These include primary central nervous system lymphoma, high-grade B-cell lymphomas, atypical Hodgkin's disease, and Kaposi sarcoma (KS). The lymphomas are covered in previous chapter in this book while the latter malignancy, KS, will be the focus of this chapter.

KS is a multifocal neoplasm of unknown etiology that arises from lymphatic endothelial cells. It was the first cancer to be associated with AIDS and is the most common neoplasm that occurs in HIV-infected persons [1,2]. At one time, it was reported in up to 40% of reported cases of AIDS, but the incidence has decreased to 14% of all reported cases [3]. Although AIDS-related KS has been reported among all risk groups for AIDS, 95% of cases have occurred among homosexual/bisexual men with AIDS. The male-to-female ratio is 50:1. Women are more likely to have KS if their partners are bisexual men than if they are intravenous drug abusers, supporting the observation that KS usually results from sexual contact rather than parenteral transmission.

Multiple factors may increase the prevalence of KS in HIV infection. These include defects in both cellular and humoral mechanisms of immune surveillance, the presence of viruses that may cause malignant transformation, and dysregulated B-cell and monocyte stimulation. KS is clinically aggressive and displays unusual patterns of organ involvement in the setting of AIDS, involving multiple organs including the gastrointestinal tract, lungs, lymph nodes, mucous membranes, skin, liver, spleen, and bone. KS is refractory to conventional therapy that is usually successful in immunocompetent patients [5,6].

Although immune deficiency is not necessary for the development of KS, it is postulated as a risk factor that can lead to KS. This idea is supported by the appearance of KS in patients with renal transplants who are treated with immunosuppressive therapy followed by regression of the tumor when the therapy is discontinued [7,8].

Three forms of KS have been described: a classic form, an aggressive form, and an AIDS-related form. The classic form is seen mainly in Eastern European and Italian men over the age of 50, where it behaves as an indolent neoplasm producing violaceous cutaneous lesions on the lower extremities [6,9,10]. An aggressive form has been described in equatorial Africa with involvement of the gastrointestinal tract, lymph nodes, gingival mucosa, and bone [10,11]. These patients tend to be younger than those with conventional KS (mean age of 41 years), they are more commonly female (3:1 female-to-male ratio, compared with more than 10:1 for classic KS), and they are of a better socioeconomic status [12]. The osseous involvement in this form of KS is usually characterized by erosion of bone by adjacent cutaneous lesions. There is often osseous destruction, cortical erosion, and periosteal reaction. Kyalwazi described two patterns of osseous abnormality in this form of KS: histologically negative discrete pressure erosions on bone from overlying soft tissue lesions and histologically positive osteoporosis progressing to destruction, associated with the infiltrative clinical pattern [13]. An AIDS-related form of KS has now been described in HIV-positive patients which more closely resembles the aggressive African form.

AIDS-related KS differs from the classical form of KS in many ways. The average age of 34 years in AIDS-KS patients is much lower than the average age of the patient with classical KS. The tumor is also more widespread in the AIDS-related form. Lesions of KS can develop at any time during the course of HIV infection. Involvement of the skin is usually seen on the arms, head and neck, and trunk, with occasional involvement of the lower extremities [14].

Histologic features of AIDS-KS include lymphatic and vascular proliferation, mononuclear cell infiltration, and spindle cell formation [6]. The tumor can have a varied clinical course. The most common presentation is a rapid fulminant course with extensive involvement of the skin and visceral organs. There is also a small group of patients who have had indolent disease for many years. Average median survival time for patients with AIDS-KS is related to the T-cell count and constitutional symptoms and ranges from 14-32 months [15].

Scintigraphy can be used to evaluate patients with suspected KS. Cutaneous lesions of KS demonstrate increased RBC pooling on Technetium-99m-MDP labeled red blood cell imaging, increased Thallium-201 uptake, and absent Gallium uptake, contrary to infections and other tumors, which demonstrate increased Gallium uptake [16].

Treatment of KS varies according to symptoms and the site of involvement. The painful osseous lesions, which are described later in this chapter, were irradiated, with symptomatic relief. Treatment of symptomatic or cosmetically troublesome skin lesions involves resection, irradiation, liquid nitrogen cryotherapy or electrocautery, and intralesional administration of vincristine sulfate, vinblastine sulfate, bleomycin, or interferon-alpha. Interferon is the treatment of choice over chemotherapy when systemic treatment is necessary.

Until recently, there were only two case reports describing bone marrow involvement in patients with AIDS-related KS [17,18]. No direct biopsies of osseous lesions had been performed. Subsequently, we reported two patients with biopsy proven KS of bone [19]. In one patient, there were multiple osteolytic lesions located in the pelvis, hips, ribs, and spine. The other patient had focal permeative destruction of the proximal humeral diaphysis which also extended to the shoulder joint, where there was an osseous erosion and an effusion.

CASE STUDIES

Two men in our patient population had biopsy-proven osseous involvement secondary to KS.

Case 1

This patient was a 33-year-old man who presented with known Kaposi sarcoma of the skin, lung, and abdominal and pelvic nodes. On conventional radiographs there were multiple lytic lesions in the ribs (Fig. l-A) and pelvis. CT demonstrated multiple discrete lytic lesions in the lumbar spine and iliac crests (Fig. l-B& C). Technetium-99m-MDP whole-body scintigrams obtained at the time of the radiographs and CT demonstrated only focal abnormalities in the skull, manubrium, and the right costochondral junction of the tenth rib (Fig. l-D). No areas of abnormal tracer uptake were found in the spine, pelvis or right femur in the region of the lytic lesions. A Gallium-67 citrate scan also failed to demonstrate any lesions in the skeleton. The lesions did not heal with doxycycline antibiotic therapy. A biopsy of a lesion in the iliac crest was consistent with KS (Fig. l-E). There was no evidence of bacillary angiomatosis on Warthin-Starry stain. The patient was treated with radiation and chemotherapy.

Case 2

The other patient was a 43-year-old man with known diffuse cutaneous Kaposi sarcoma, diagnosed one and one-half years prior to involvement of his right shoulder with the disease. He developed sudden onset of shoulder pain and had a normal conventional shoulder radiograph. CT obtained three weeks later demonstrated medullary destruction and cortical erosions of the anterior and

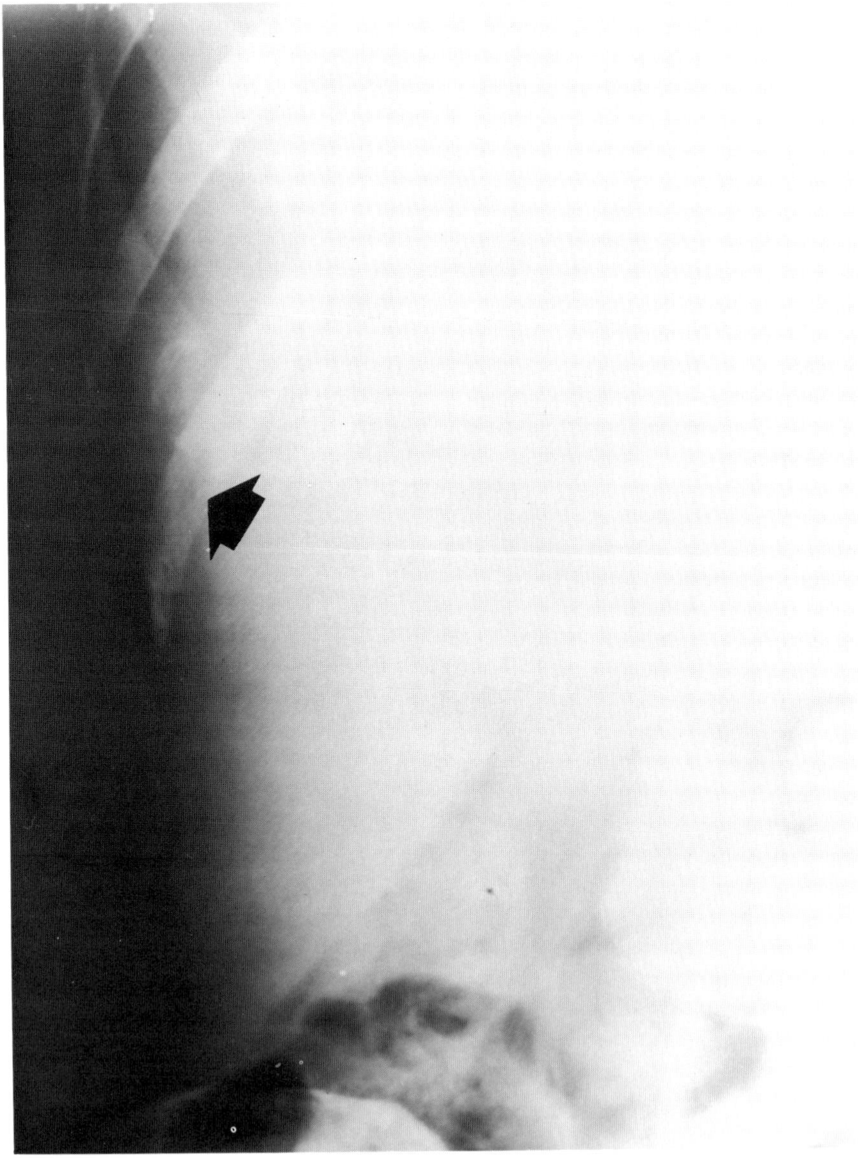

Figure 1-A

Multifocal skeletal Kaposi sarcoma. This patient with biopsy-proven KS of bone had multiple lytic lesions throughout the bones. A lytic lesion was seen in the right eleventh rib on conventional radiographs (arrow).

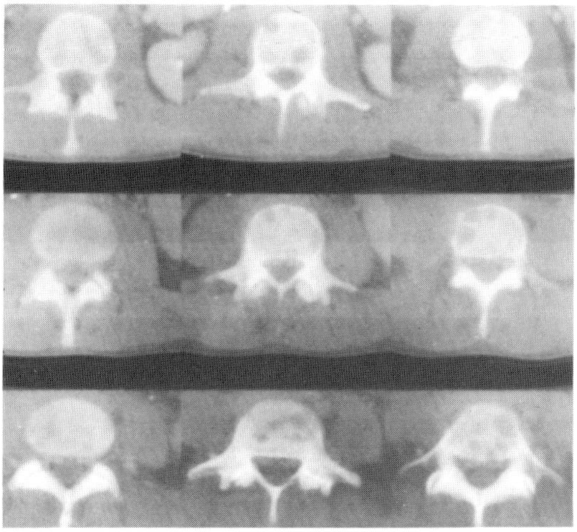

Figure 1-B
There are multiple focal lytic lesions within the lumbar vertebral bodies, demonstrated on consecutive images of the lumbar spine.

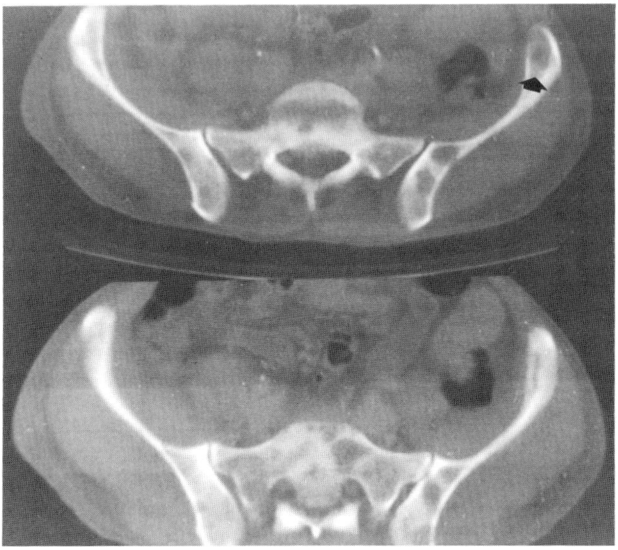

Figure 1-C
Two consecutive CT images through the iliac crests demonstrate lytic lesions in both ilii and sacrum. A biopsy of the large lesion in the left iliac crest (arrow) was consistent with Kaposi sarcoma.

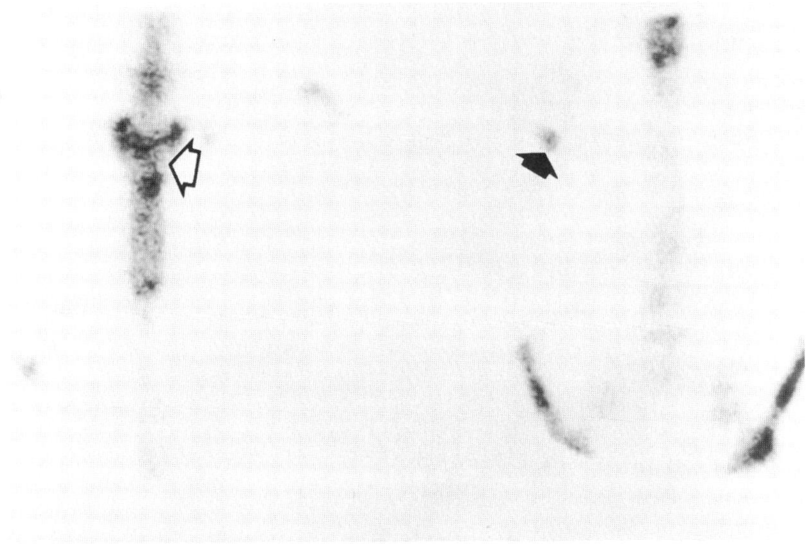

Figure 1-D
A Technetium-99m-MDP whole-body scintigram demonstrates high uptake in the costochondral junction of the tenth rib (black arrow) and the sternomanubrial area (open arrow). The lytic lesions seen on CT in the spine and iliac crests are not visualized on the scan.

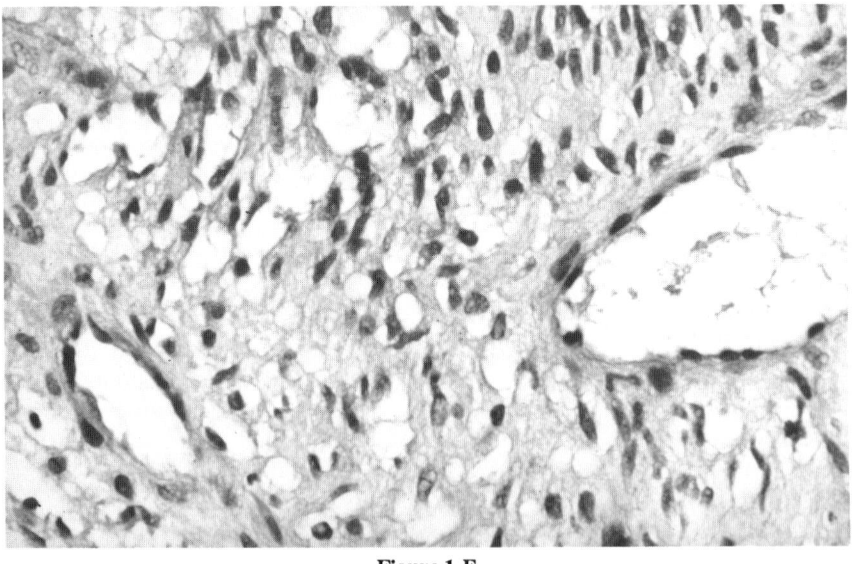

Figure 1-E
A biopsy of the lesion in the left iliac crest demonstrates numerous hyperchromatic spindled cells forming fascicles, consistent with Kaposi sarcoma.

posterolateral surfaces of the humeral head (Fig. 2-A). MRI obtained at the same time showed focal abnormal signal intensity, noted centrally in the proximal humeral head and shaft (Fig. 2-B,C&D). There was also an effusion in the shoulder joint. A bone biopsy of the humeral head was consistent with KS. A Warthin-Starry stain for bacillary angiomatosis was negative. The shoulder was treated with radiation therapy (2,500 rads in 10 fractions), which provided symptomatic relief.

OBSERVATIONS

It has been shown previously that skin involvement precedes most cases of pulmonary KS. As with pulmonary KS, in the two patients we encountered with skeletal KS, the osseous lesions developed after the appearance of skin lesions.

A Technetium-99m-MDP bone scan was obtained and failed to detect many of the osseous lesions in the first patient, whose case history is recounted here as well as in the patient with osseous KS described by Meyers [18]. Therefore, it appears that radiographs, CT or MRI of the symptomatic areas should be obtained for early detection of osseous KS lesions in patients with known KS who have bone pain. The Gallium scan was also negative in the first patient described here (Case 1), similar to observations disclosed in other studies [16,20]. These patterns on scintigraphy may aid in distinguishing KS from infections such as bacillary angiomatosis, which may be detected on bone scintigraphy and/or Gallium scan prior to demonstration by conventional radiography [21]. Osseous lesions of KS have a similar appearance to other types of osseous lesions that have been described in AIDS patients, including infections such as bacillary angiomatosis, tuberculosis, and fungus, as well as lymphoma. In fact, many HIV-positive patients with KS have these other diseases as well, therefore, it is imperative to biopsy these lesions so that appropriate treatment may be initiated. A Warthin-Starry stain is usually performed to exclude bacillary angiomatosis. Especially in this patient population, delay in treatment or inappropriate treatment can be detrimental, if not fatal. Infections should be treated with antibiotics, whereas lymphoma and KS are usually treated with removal of the lesion, radiation, interferon, and/or chemotherapy. The osseous lesions of KS described in this report were treated with radiation, which provided symptomatic relief.

CONCLUSION

KS is relatively frequent in the HIV-positive patient population. Skeletal lesions of KS are rare, with only four reported cases. Even though skeletal involvement is unusual, one should consider KS in patients who are HIV-positive who present with lytic or permeative lesions of bone. More common

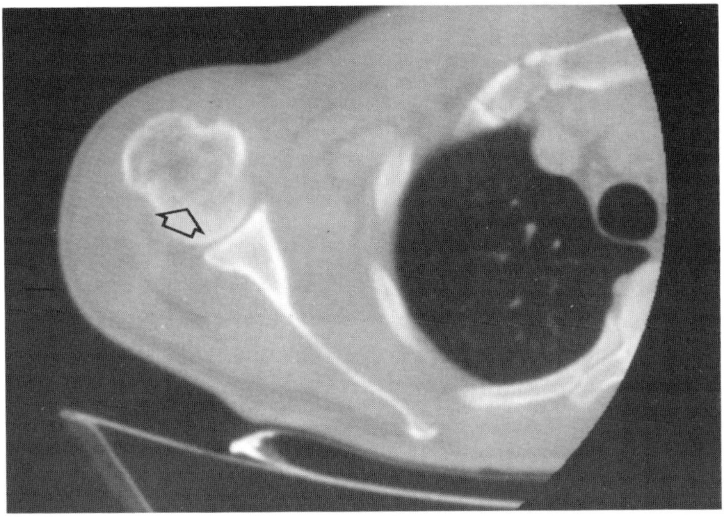

Figure 2-A.

Multifocal skeletal Kaposi sarcoma. Kaposi sarcoma of the humeral head and shoulder. CT of the right humeral head obtained at the time of CT-guided biopsy reveals permeative lytic destruction of the medullary space (arrow). Posterolateral cortical disruption was present on more proximal CT images of the humeral head and is also demonstrated on MRI in Figure 2-B.

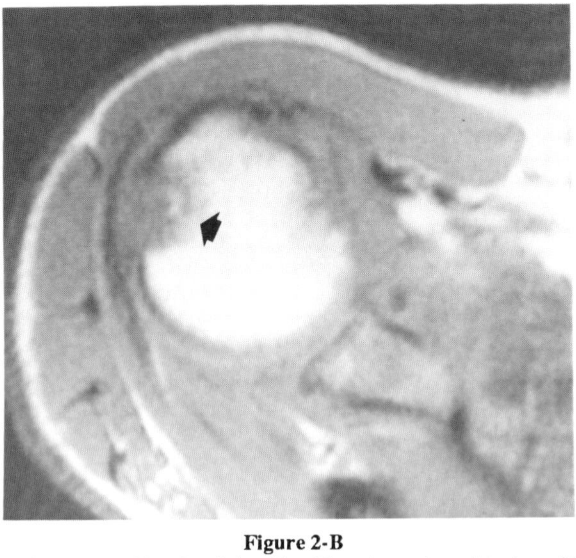

Figure 2-B

Kaposi sarcoma of the humeral head and shoulder. There is erosion of the lateral humeral head on this axial Tl-weighted (TR=700, TE=12) MR image of the shoulder joint (arrow).

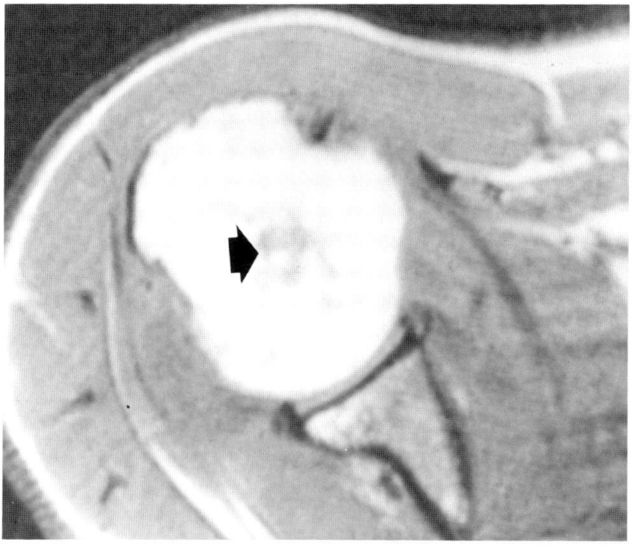

Figure 2-C

Axial Tl-weighted image obtained further caudally reveals an abnormal low signal intensity lesion within the high signal intensity marrow (arrow).

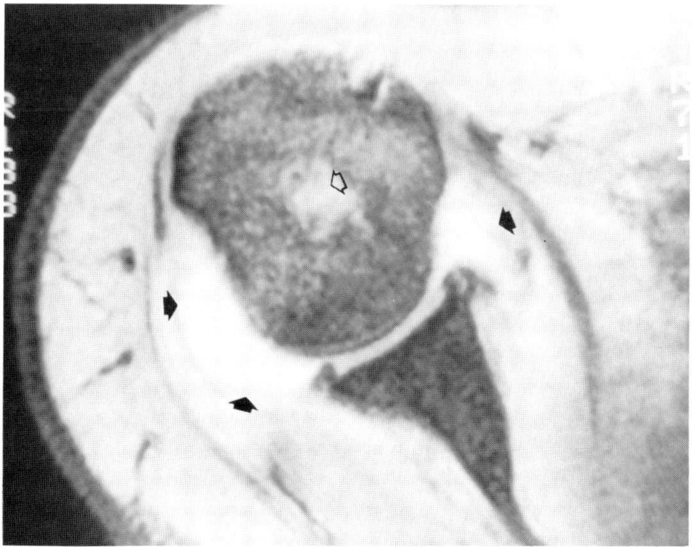

Figure 2-D

The lesion increases in signal intensity on a corresponding gradient echo MR image (TR=400, TE=15, flip angle=20) (open arrow). There is also a large high signal intensity effusion in the shoulder joint which is distending the anterior and posterior capsule (black arrows).

abnormalities such as osteomyelitis secondary to common bacteria or opportunistic organisms, tuberculosis, fungal disease, bacillary angiomatosis, and lymphoma should also be considered. If the lesion does not respond to antibiotic therapy, biopsy of the lesion is recommended to ensure prompt and appropriate treatment.

REFERENCES

1. Haverkos HV, Friedman-Kien AE, Drotman DP, Morgan WM. The changing incidence of Kaposi's sarcoma among patients with AIDS. *J Am Acad Dermatol* 1990;22:1250-1253.
2. Rabkin CS, Biggar RJ, Horm JW. Increasing incidence of cancers associated with the human immunodeficiency virus epidemic. *Int J Cancer* 1991;47:692-696.
3. Friedman-Kien AE, Saltzman BR. Clinical manifestations of classical, endemic African and endemic AIDS-associated Kaposi's sarcoma. *J Am Acad Dermatol* 1990;22:1237-1250.
4. Centers for Disease Control. Revision of the case definition of acquired immunodeficiency syndrome for national reporting - United States. *MMWR* 1985;34:373-375.
5. Groopman JE, Broder S. Cancers in AIDS and other immunodeficiency states. In: DeVita VT, Hellan S, Rosenberg SA (eds), *Cancer Principles and Practice of Oncology,* 3rd ed. Philadelphia: J.B. Lippincott, 1989,1953-1970.
6. Safai B, Schwartz JJ, Dias BM. Malignant neoplasms associated with human immunodeficiency virus infection. *Ca Cancer J Clin* 1992;42:74-75.
7. Pilgrim M. Spontaneous manifestation and regression of a Kaposi's sarcoma under cyclosporin. *A Hautarzt* 1988;39:368-370.
8. Wijnveen AC, Persson H, Bjorck S, Dlohme I. Disseminated Kaposi's sarcoma: full regression after withdrawal of immunosuppressive therapy: report of a case. *Transplant Proc* 1987;19:3735-3736.
9. Mitsuyasi RT. Kaposi's sarcoma in the acquired immunodeficiency syndrome. *Infect Dis Clin North Am* 1988;2:511-523.
10. Taylor JF, Templeton AC, Vogel CL, Ziegler JL, Kyalwazi SK. Kaposi's sarcoma in Uganda: a clinico-pathological study. *Int J Cancer* 1971;8:122-135.
11. Bayley AC. Atypical aggressive Kaposi's sarcoma in Africa. In: Gottlieg GJ, Ackerman B (eds), *Kaposi's Sarcoma: A Text and Atlas.* Philadelphia: Lea and Febiger, 1981, 151-170.
12. Bayley AC. Aggressive Kaposi's sarcoma in Zambia: 1983. *Lancet* 1984;1:1318.
13. Kyalwazi SK. Kaposi's sarcoma: clinical features, experience in Uganda. *Antibiot Chemother* 1981;29:59.
14. Safai B, Johnson KG, Myskowski PL, et al. The natural history of Kaposi's sarcoma in the acquired immunodeficiency syndrome. *Ann Int Med* 1985;103:744-750.

15. Chachoua A, Krigel R, Lafleur F, et al. Prognostic factors and staging classification of patients with epidemic Kaposi's sarcoma. *J Clin Oncol* 1989;7:774-780.
16. Vanarthos WJ, Ganz WI, Vanarthos JC, Serafini AN, Tehranzadeh J. Diagnostic uses of nuclear medicine in AIDS. *RadioGraphics* 1992;12:731-749.
17. Little BJ, Spivak JL, Quinn TC, Mann RB. Case report: Kaposi's sarcoma with bone marrow involvement: occurrence in a patient with acquired immunodeficiency syndrome. *Am I Med Sci* 1986;292:44-46.
18. Meyers SA, Kuhlman JE, Fishman EK. Kaposi sarcoma involving bone: CT demonstration in a patient with AIDS. *J Comput Assist Tomogr* 1990;14:161-162.
19. Steinbach LS, Tehranzadeh J, Fleckenstein JL, Vanarthos W, Pais MJ. Human immunodeficiency virus: musculoskeletal manifestations. *Radiology* 1993;186:833-838.
20. Lee VW, Fuller JD, O'Brien MJ, et al. Pulmonary Kaposi sarcoma in patients with AIDS: scintigraphic diagnosis with sequential thallium and gallium scanning. *Radiology* 1991;180:409.
21. Baron AL, Steinbach LS, LeBoit PE, Mills CM, Gee JH, Berger TG. Osteolytic lesions and bacillary angiomatosis in HIV infection: radiologic differentiation from AIDS-related Kaposi sarcoma. *Radiology* 1990;177:77-81.

CHAPTER 8:

BONE MARROW ABNORMALITIES IN AIDS PATIENTS

Jamshid Tehranzadeh, M.D.
Chris Cassady, M.D.

The majority of reported cases of AIDS with bone marrow involvement have been secondary to common focal infection, unusual opportunistic pathogens, and tumoral growth, primarily high-grade lymphomas and sarcoma. Extensive changes in hematopoietic function affecting marrow composition in the axial and appendicular skeleton are also well described though, to date, their description in imaging studies remains limited.

Hematopoietic dysfunction in HIV-infected patients may have multiple etiologies. HIV itself causes suppression of growth in myeloid and erythroid cell lines in vitro (1). Studies suggest that HIV can directly infect both marrow cells and their precursors and that there may be soluble products inhibiting hematopoiesis in infected individuals (2). Pathogens, including infection and malignancy, and their chemotherapeutic treatments are also implicated in myelosuppression. Marrow biopsy samples have demonstrated an incidence of myelodysplasia of nearly 70% in one series (3). Serous fat atrophy, a condition noted previously to occur in patients with severe malnutrition and weight loss, has also been seen (9-39%).

A retrospective examination of the bone marrow biopsies performed by Banez et al (4) in 61 consecutive patients with acquired immune deficiency syndrome showed hypercellularity in 76% of the cases, increased myeloid/erythroid (ME) ratio in 35%, increased megakariocytes in 50%, plasmacytosis in 36%, fibrosis in 90%, and increased iron stores in 77%. Lymphohistiocytic proliferation was observed in 38%. Thirty percent (30%) had granulomas. Acid fast bacilli were demonstrated in 11%, and fungi in 10%.

Peripheral anemia in HIV-infected individuals is endemic(5). A normochromic/normocytic erythroid pattern with a suppression of reticulocytosis is typical. Previously, this was seen in association with various inflammatory and autoimmune processes, and has been termed the anemia of chronic disease (6). In a study by Karcher (3) of over 200 biopsies from patients with AIDS, 65% of the samples demonstrated evidence of reticuloendothelial iron blockade, a dysfunction involving impaired release of iron from marrow macrophages, resulting in low serum iron and total iron-binding capacity but an elevation in marrow iron stores. RE blockade has generally been associated with the anemia of chronic disease. In Karcher's study, the pattern correlates with CDC class IV disease and is strongly associated with a history of opportunistic infections.

This RE blockade has been proposed by Geremia et al as the source of diffuse hypointensive marrow change on magnetic resonance imaging of the spine in AIDS patients (7). The usual appearance of higher signal intensity vertebral bodies adjacent to lower signal intensity intervertebral discs is inverted on T1-weighted images in some AIDS patients, a finding that tends to be diffuse throughout all levels of the spine. Both homogeneous and, less often, mottled heterogeneous hypointensity on T1-weighted images can mimic changes seen with infiltrating tumor of the bone marrow. T2-weighted images remain unaffected.

Marrow in the vertebral body of a normal control gives it an appearance equal to or brighter than the intervertebral discs with Tl-weighting. In the average young adult, cellular marrow is composed of approximately 40% fat by weight; an increase with aging to 60-80% fat is expected (8). Fat tends to shorten T1 relaxation time on magnetic resonance images and consequently appears bright. Changes in marrow signal theoretically may reflect alterations in marrow composition, including fat/myeloid ratio variability or the introduction of abnormal amounts of other paramagnetic substances. Although fat/myeloid ratios may be highly variable in AIDS patients, this has not been shown to correlate with imaging changes (7).

In the series reported by Steinbach et al (9), five men had hypointense marrow incidentally demonstrated on MR images of the spine that had been obtained because of neck or back pain. These patients ranged in age from 30 to 48 years. The marrow had lower signal intensity than the discs with all imaging sequences, including a T1weighted (500/20) sequence (Figs. 1-3).

Paramagnetic hemosiderin in the iron-laden macrophages seen with RE blockade may be responsible for the T1 marrow signal inversion. An increased volume of ferric iron shortens both T1 and T2 relaxation times but the effect is a relative one; changes to normal marrow signal are moderate on T1 but less noticeable with T2-weighted images, where marrow is already of low signal.

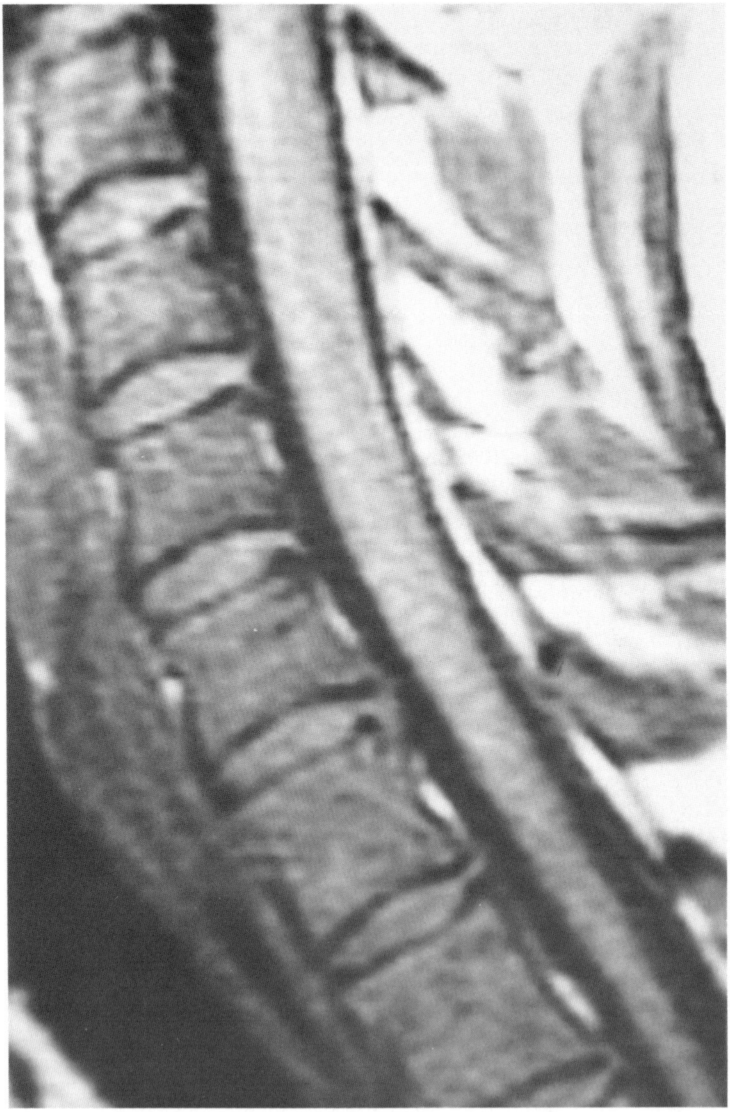

Figure 1-A

Hypointense marrow. Hypointense marrow in the cervical spine of a 30-year-old male with HIV infection. (From Steinbach LS: *Radiology* 1993;186:833-838, with permission). Sagittal T1WI (TR/TE 600/11) shows diffuse hypointensity throughout the vertebral bodies on this image. The marrow is of lower signal intensity than the disc, a finding that can be seen with hemosiderosis from anemia of chronic disease.

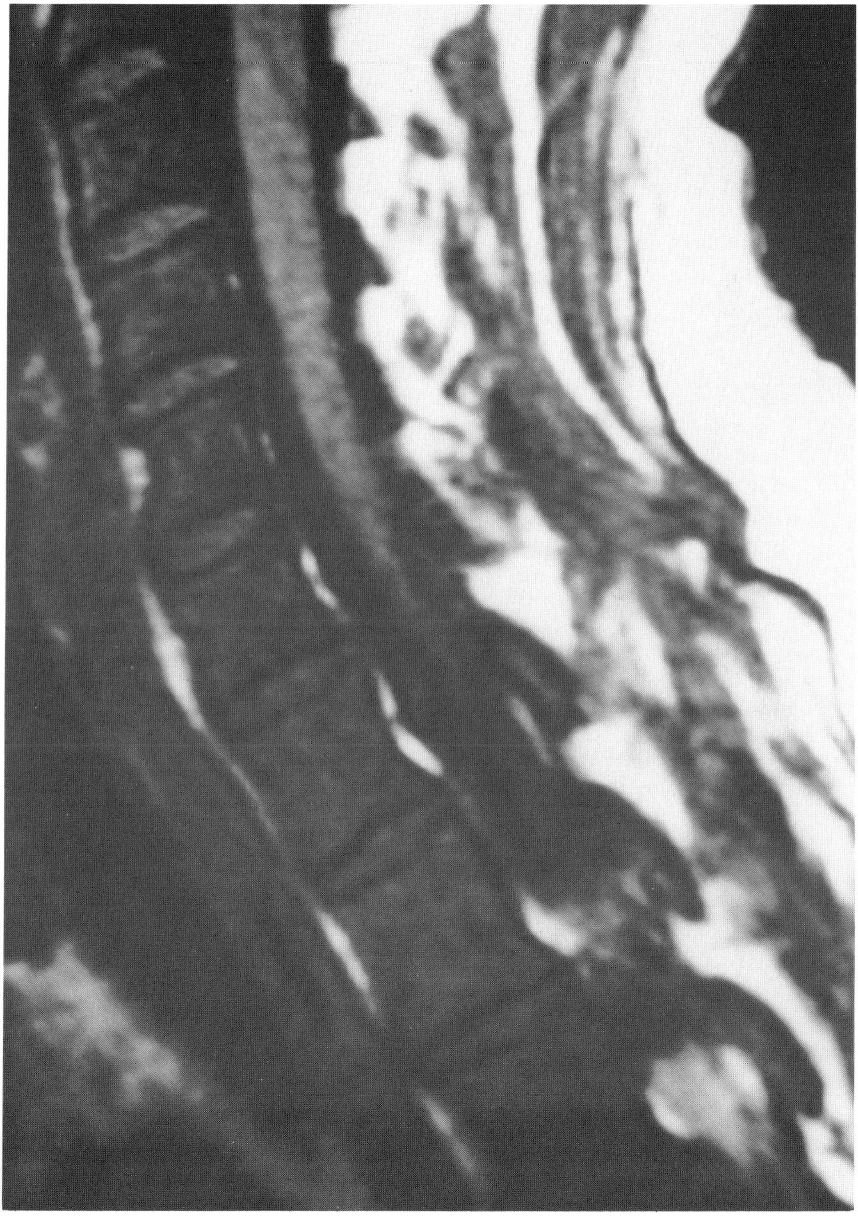

Figure 1-B

Sagittal T1WI (TR/TE 600/20) of the cervical spine (same patient as 1-A) shows diffuse hypointense marrow throughout the cervical spine.

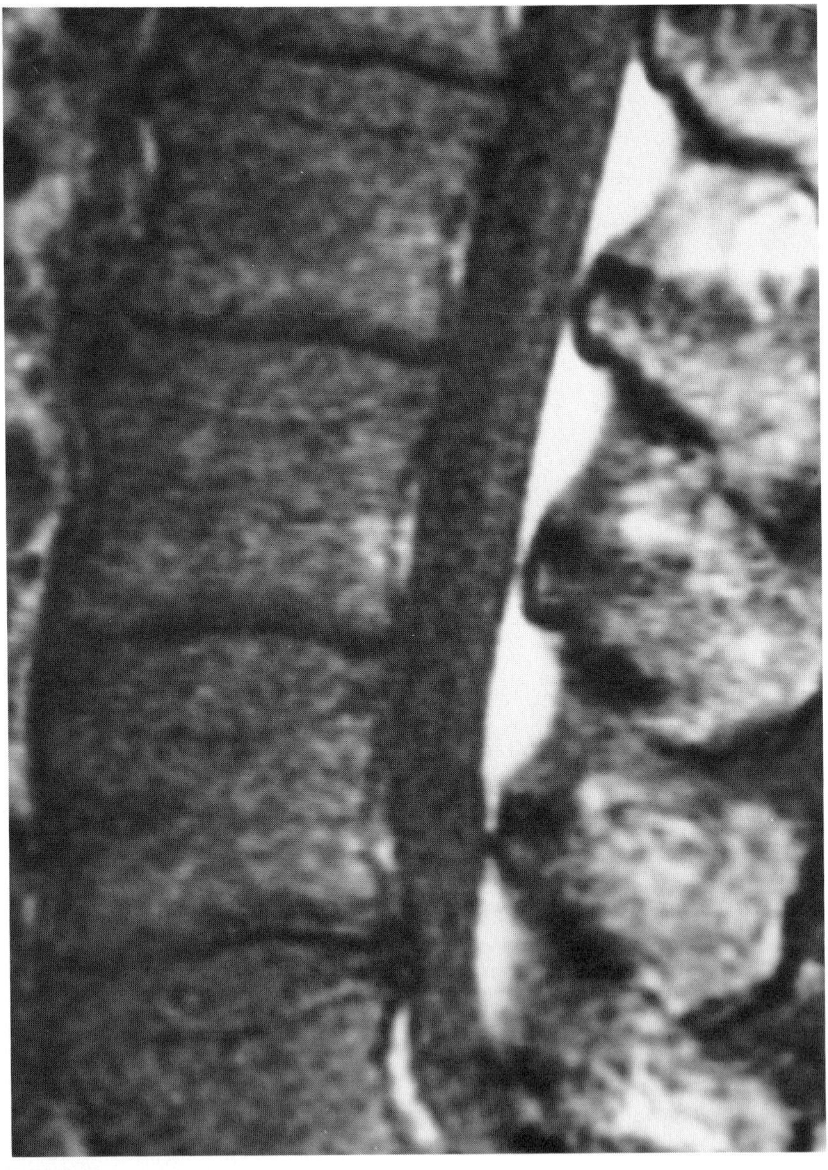

Figure 2

Hypointense marrow. Hypointense marrow in the lumbar spine in a 48-year-old black male with HIV infection. The marrow is diffusely hypointense throughout the vertebral bodies on this sagittal T1WI (TR/TE 500/20) image.

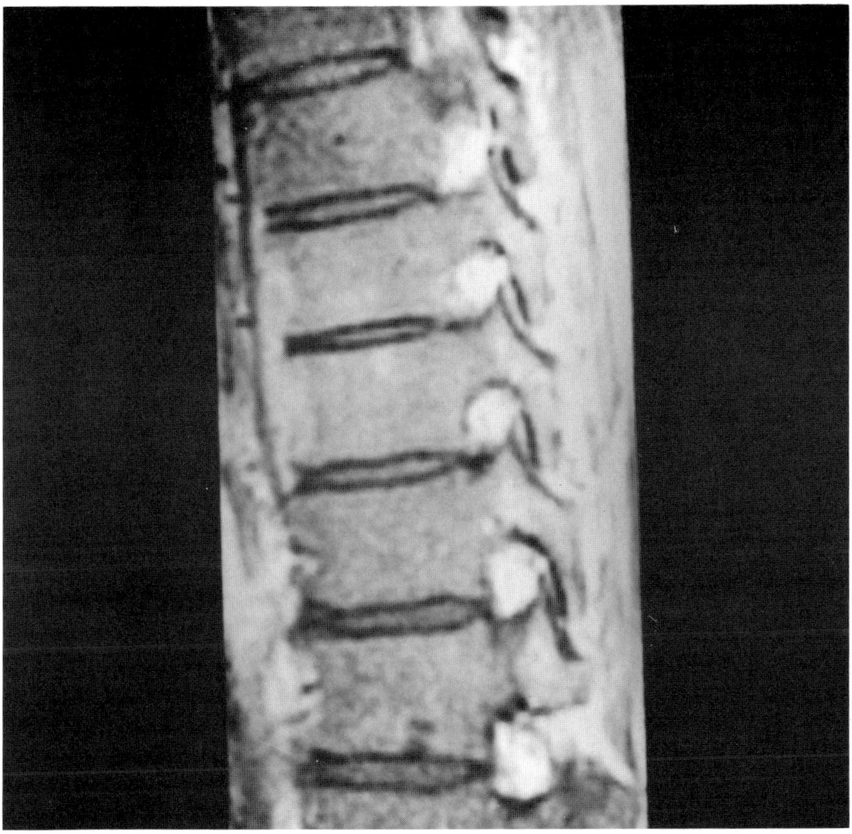

Figure 3

Hypointense marrow. 48-year-old male physician with HIV infection. Sagittal TlWI (TR/TR 500/12) of thoracic spine with intravenous Gadolinium shows diffuse hypointensity of bone marrow. Note that marrow signal intensity is less than that of the intervertebral disc, even on this enhanced T1-weighted image.

Patients may have localizable pain as the indication for examinations but in many cases the finding is incidental, noted in the cervical spine during examination of the brain or in the lumbar spine during a pelvis study. Clinical circumstances and the wide extent of involvement help differentiate the MR reflection of diffuse marrow dysfunction and associated RE blockade from infiltrative disease, such as infection or tumor. It is unclear whether this effect plays any role in the imaging of pediatric patients with HIV, in whom marrow signal varies in intensity due to a relative hypercellularity in children (8,10).

REFERENCES

1. Steinberg HN, Crumpacker CS, Chatis PA. In vitro suppression of normal human bone marrow progenitor cells by human immunodeficiency virus. *J Virology* 1991 Apr;65(4):1765-1769.
2. Aboulafia DM, Mitsuyasu RT. Hematologic abnormalities in AIDS. *Hemat/Oncol Clin North Am* 1991 Apr;5(2):195-214.
3. Karcher DS, Prost AR. The bone marrow in human immunodeficiency virus (HIV)-related disease. Morphology and clinical correlation. *Am J Clin Pathol* 1991 Jan;95(1):63-71.
4. Banez EI, Ansari MQ. Is the bone marrow examination useful in the investigation of the acquired immunodeficiency syndrome? Presented at the 82nd Annual Scientific Meeting of the Southern Medical Association, November 6-9,1988.
5. Harris CE, Biggs JC, Concannon AJ, Dodds AJ. Peripheral blood and bone marrow findings in patients with acquired immune deficiency syndrome. *Pathology* 1990 Oct;22(4):206-211.
6. Cartwright C. The anemia of chronic disorders. *Semin Hematol* 1966;3:351-375.
7. Geremia GK, McCluney KW, Adler SS, et al. The magnetic resonance hypointense spine of AIDS. *J Comput Assist Tomogr* 1990 Sept/Oct;14(5):785-789.
8. Steiner RM, Mitchell DG, Rao VM, Murphy S, Rifkin MD, Burk DL Jr, Vinitski S. Magnetic resonance imaging of bone marrow: diagnostic value in diffuse hematologic disorders. *Magn Res Quar* 1990 Jan;6(1):17-34.
9. Steinbach LS, Tehranzadeh J, Fleckenstein JL, Vanarthos WJ, Pais MJ. Human immunodeficiency virus infection: musculoskeletal manifestations. *Radiology* 1993;186:833-838.
10. Sandhaus LM, Scudder R. Hematologic and bone marrow abnormalities in pediatric patients with human immunodeficiency virus (HIV) infection. *Pediatr Pathol* 1989;9:277-288.

CHAPTER 9:

MISCELLANEOUS MUSCULOSKELETAL CONDITIONS ASSOCIATED WITH HIV INFECTION

Jamshid Tehranzadeh, M.D.
Chris Cassady, M.D.

Common pathologic entities associated with infection by the human immunodeficiency virus and involving the musculoskeletal system have been discussed and their imaging findings presented. The characteristic features of several related processes have been cited in connection with HIV infection on a more sporadic basis. These conditions can be categorized as follows:

A. *Systemic Changes*
   1. Multiple myeloma
   2. Skeletal metastasis
   3. Osteonecrosis
   4. Necrotizing periodontitis
   5. Myopathy
   6. Myositis ossificans

B. *Peripheral Skeletal Changes*
   1. Hypertrophic osteoarthropathy
   2. Reflex sympathetic dystrophy
   3. Dupuytren's contracture

A. SYSTEMIC CHANGES

1. *Multiple Myeloma*

High-grade B-cell lymphomas and leukemia have been well-described in AIDS patients. Multiple myeloma and extramedullary plasmacytomas are rarely reported but remain a consideration in patients with monoclonal gammopathy or osteolytic bone lesions (1-5). Multiple myeloma in AIDS is all the more striking for its development in younger persons. The immune dysregulation of HIV may allow for increased susceptibility of well-differentiated B-lymphocytes to malignant transformation. Additionally, retroviral infection itself directly accelerates plasmacytogenesis in vitro (6). Concurrent infection by Epstein-Barr virus may also play a pathogenic role via clonal expansion (7). Reported cases include non-secretory tumors as well as those with no evidence of osseous involvement, in addition to those cases with classic findings of solitary plasmacytoma of bone or multiple osteolytic lesions (8-10).

2. *Skeletal Metastasis*

We have encountered a single case of metastatic adenocarcinoma in an HIV-positive patient with an expansile lytic lesion of the left ilium. A primary site of the cancer was never identified in this case (Fig. 1).

3. *Osteonecrosis*

Avascular necrosis (AVN) of bone, or osteonecrosis, has generally been associated with trauma, chronic systemic disease which can cause vascular flow disruption, or long-term use of agents known to increase marrow lipid volume with a theoretical increase in intramedullary pressures and arterial occlusion

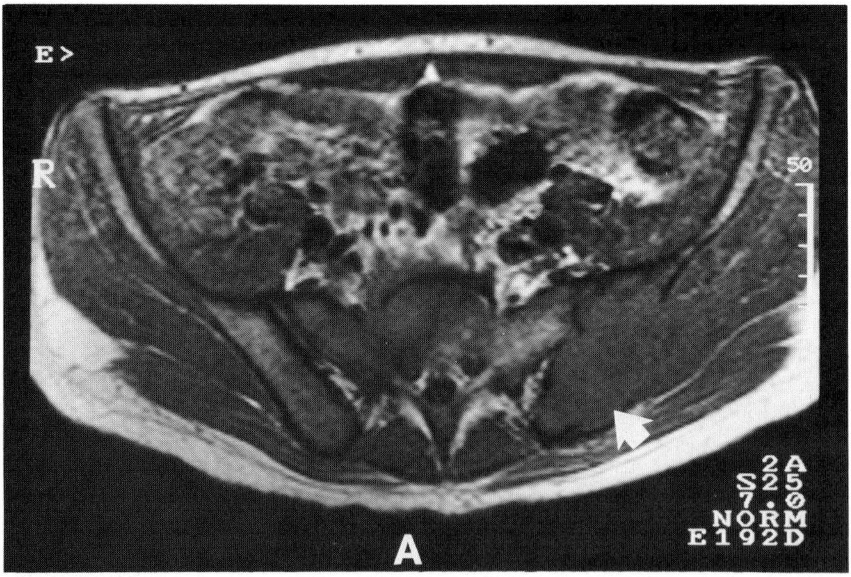

Figure 1-A

Metastatic adenocarcinoma. HIV-positive patient with metastatic adenocarcinoma. (Courtesy of James L. Fleckenstein). Axial T1-weighted image (TR 500/TE 15) (A), proton density (TR 2000/TE 30) (B), T2-weighted image (TR 2000/TE 100) (C) and STIR 2000/30/150 (TR/TE/TI) (D) images of pelvis show large expansile lesion of the left ilium with soft tissue extension into the left buttock, well demonstrated on each sequence (arrow). A CT-guided biopsy revealed metastatic adenocarcinoma.

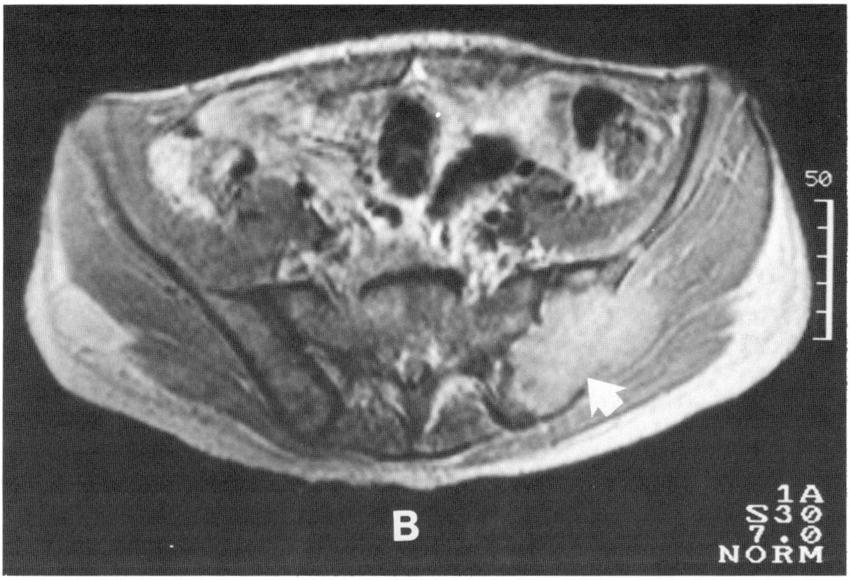

Figure 1-B

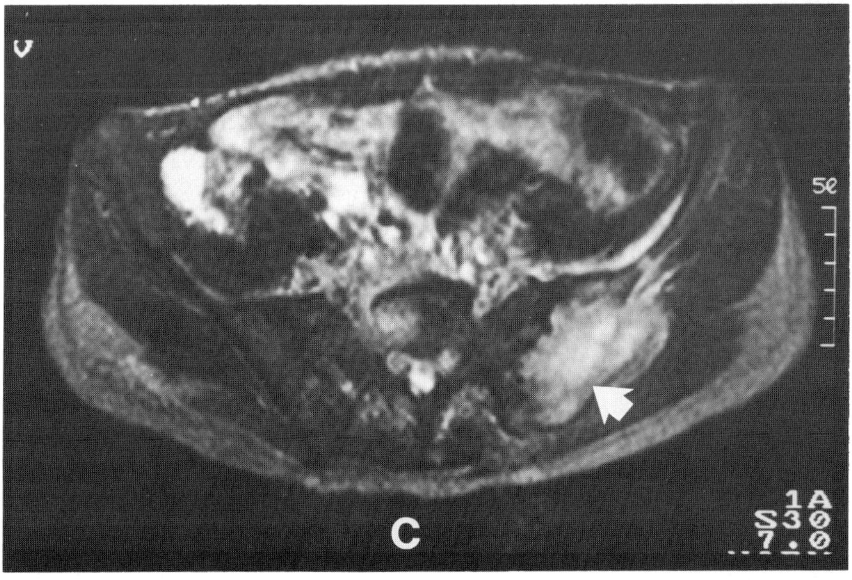

Figure 1-C

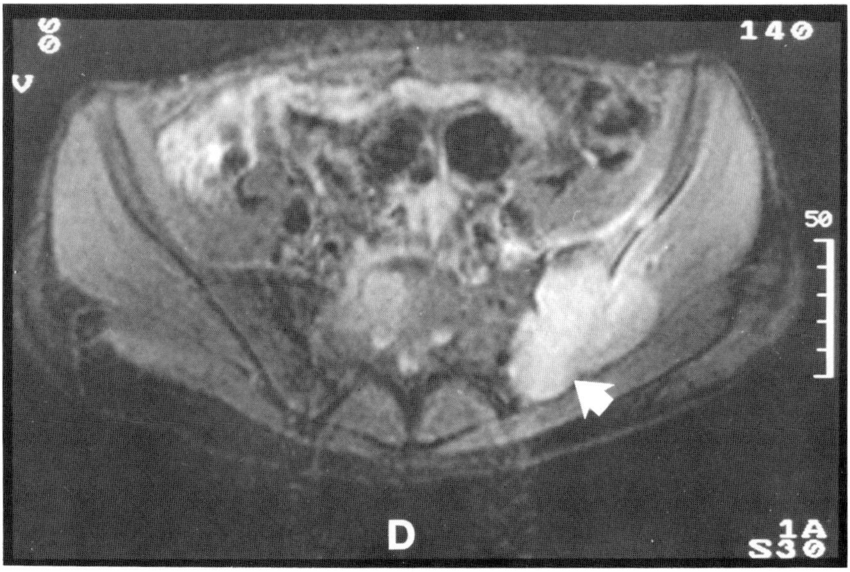

Figure 1-D

(11,12). The AVN etiology may also be unknown in many cases though its presence at multiple sites has been particularly related to hypercortisonism (13). However, HIV may be an additional cause of single or multiple site involvement by AVN, as several reports suggest (Fig. 2) (14-16). Circulatory disruption as a result of underlying vasculitis, an inflammatory state not uncommon in AIDS patients, is postulated as a mechanism for the development of AVN (17).

Plain film findings in the hips and shoulders are classic for AVN. Subchondral fracture with a curvilinear or "crescentic" radiolucency can be followed by development of sclerotic and rarefied cystic foci in the epiphysis during attempts at repair. Irreversible manifestations include flattening of the epiphyseal head, widening of the epiphyseal line and rarefaction of the metaphysis. Joint spaces remain preserved. Magnetic resonance imaging is highly sensitive to early AVN, showing heterogeneous changes in signal in affected areas, reflecting both the extent of the lesion and the stage of the disease. High signal intensity with T1- and low signal intensity with T2-weighting predominates early, reversing as edema increases and the lesion progresses. A "double line" sign may be present with a thick band of decreased signal intensity marginating the lesion on T1-weighted images. T2-weighted images show a second adjacent inner band of increased intensity. These appear secondary to both changes in marrow composition and chemical shift artifact (18). In addition, the merits of bone scintigraphy in the evaluation of AVN are well-described (19).

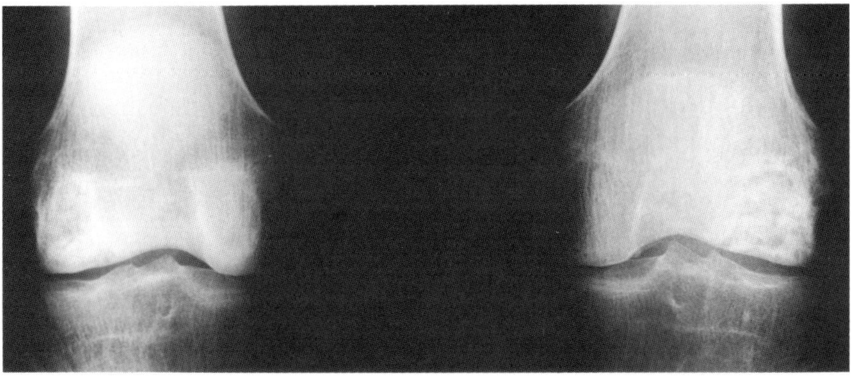

Figure 2-A

Osteonecrosis. Osteonecrosis of femoral condyles in a 34-year-old HIV-positive man with meningitis. AP view of both knees shows osteonecrosis of femoral condyles of both knees.

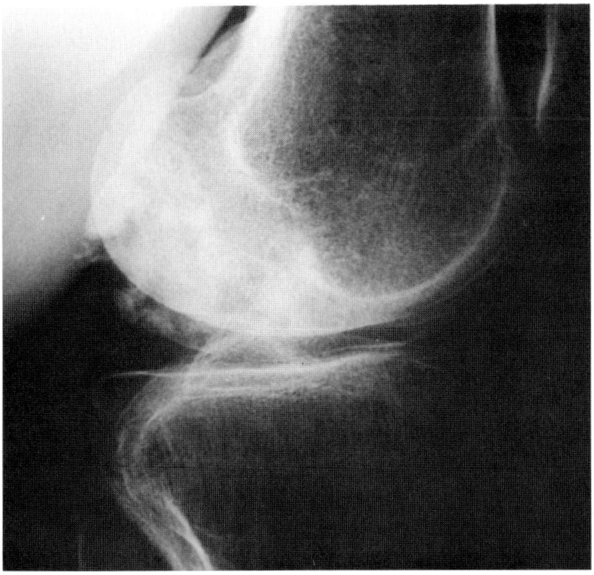

Figure 2-B

Lateral view of the left knee shows osteonecrosis with subchondral fracture and fragmentation.

4. *Necrotizing Periodontitis*

A particular pattern of osseous necrosis has been cited increasingly in the dental literature in association with profound periodontal disease (20-22). Necrotizing periodontitis is not seen in HIV-seronegative patients. It is characterized by extensive soft tissue and bony destruction, which may be focal and periapical or generalized in the more markedly immunocompromised (23). Both maxilla and mandible can be involved. Although only normal oral flora is cultured, the use of penicillin appears to arrest advancement of disease (24). The direct application of cocaine in drug users with AIDS has also been reported as a cause of focal destruction of mucosa and bone (25).

5. *Myopathy*

Myopathic involvement in patients with HIV infection both in previously asymptomatic seropositive carriers and those with developed AIDS is well-known (5). Pathologic changes in skeletal muscle may be secondary to central and peripheral nervous system disease, drug toxicity, metabolic derangement, or wasting (26-35). Primary myopathies associated with AIDS are also documented, though their pathogenesis remains uncertain. Inflammatory entities such as pyomyositis and polymyositis may be consequent to reactive immune phenomena or infection by HIV and have been discussed in previous chapters (36-38). Additionally, various authors have reported finding characteristic changes of a non-inflammatory nemaline (rod body) myopathy in HIV-positive patients complaining principally of proximal muscle weakness (39-43).

Nemaline myopathy of adult onset is a slowly progressive muscular disease, often presenting later in life (40). It has been described increasingly in younger patients with HIV infection. Many do not have clinical signs of AIDS. There may be muscle wasting with symmetric proximal muscle weakness, usually involving lower extremity and neck flexors more than the upper extremities. Myalgia is common (44). Pathologically, rods composed of actin and alpha-actin are noted to form discrete collections centrally within muscle fibers. Imaging of patients with both congenital and adult-onset rod body myopathy with HIV status unknown, has shown a diffuse decrease in density of affected muscle on CT as compared with the density of muscle in simple disuse and/or neurogenic atrophy, thought typical for primary myopathic processes (45). Computed tomography demonstrates this density variation and magnetic resonance imaging confirms nonspecific patchy, fatty degeneration throughout the muscle mass (45,46). Imaging studies in HIV-positive patients, particularly those with rod body changes, are lacking.

Other pathologic findings in diseased muscle tissue of patients with AIDS include a marked increase in iron deposition (siderosis) (47). Although theoretical alterations in density on CT or MR signal are implied, radiologic correlation has yet to be documented. For further information on muscular changes in AIDS patients, please refer to chapter 4.

6. *Myositis Ossificans*

Localized myositis ossificans is a focal, non-malignant heterotopic formation of bone or cartilage in soft tissues and muscle. Its characteristics on plain film, three-phase bone scan, gallium scintigraphy, CT, MR, and even angiography have been extensively documented (48-55). Most cases are related to antecedent trauma, but it is also found in para-articular locations in patients with nervous system dysfunction, e.g. coma or paraplegia. Development of heterotopic ossification in a patient with AIDS and chronic central nervous system depression has been reported (56).

B. PERIPHERAL SKELETAL CHANGES

1. *Hypertrophic Osteoarthropathy*

Hypertrophic osteoarthropathy (HO) is a systemic condition diagnosed by a combination of clinical and roentgenographic manifestations. These include extensive periosteal new bone formation, particularly in tubular bones of distal extremities, symmetric arthritis-type changes with arthralgia in mid-extremity joints, and clubbing of the digits. Patients may complain of burning pain or deep ache relieved by elevation of limbs. The skin over affected areas is often warm, erythematous and thickened, and significant pain may be elicited by application of pressure. Occasionally, flat bones are affected as well. In rare instances, all extremities are involved.

The pathogenesis of HO as a syndrome is obscure. Circulating hormonal factors or abnormal neural stimulation have been proposed (57). It is almost universally associated with an underlying disorder, in adults most frequently of the pulmonary system. Intrathoracic neoplasm, infection and interstitial fibrotic diseases are most common, but non-pulmonary causes including inflammatory bowel disease, abdominal abscess, cirrhosis, hemoglobinopathies, and even pregnancy are not rare. In children, HO can occur with various congenital cardiac, pulmonary and hepatic conditions. The onset of HO may precede clinical evidence of the associated disorder by months (58).

Roentgenograms demonstrate subperiosteal apposition of new bone secondary to a low-grade inflammatory reaction. In early stages, subperiosteal layering is smooth and diaphyseal but with time becomes undulating and irregular, fusion to underlying cortical bone progresses, and extension to the metaphysis and epiphysis is seen (59). Radionuclide imaging with ^{99m}Tc agents reveals increased uptake and concentration of nuclide along the metaphyseal and diaphyseal cortical surfaces, corresponding to sites of histologic heterotopic bone formation (60,61). Soft tissue thickening, joint effusion and digital clubbing have also been identified radiographically in this syndrome (62). With removal of the inciting stimulus and treatment of the associated primary disorder, resolution of symptoms is prompt and roentgenographically noted new bone resorbs, depending on extent, over weeks to months.

Case reports have identified HO in association with pulmonary *Pneumocystis carinii* infection in patients with AIDS, as well as in a patient with no demonstrable primary focus beyond his HIV status (63-65). Treatment of underlying infection provided resolution of findings in the former.

2. *Reflex Sympathetic Dystrophy*

Reflex sympathetic dystrophy syndrome, a rare condition in which localized autonomic dysfunction in a portion of an extremity is associated with Sudeck's osteoporosis, has been reported in conjunction with AIDS (66). Symptoms consist of hyperalgesia or hyperpathia with alterations in local blood flow, sweating, and hair or nail growth. There may be edema or atrophy of the skin. Roentgenographically, there is evidence of progressive and pronounced osteoporosis. It is postulated in some cases that the syndrome may be secondary to central nervous system involvement by HIV (66).

3. *Dupuytren's Contracture*

Dupuytren's contracture is shortening, thickening and fibrosis of the palmar fascia, producing a flexion deformity of a finger. An increased incidence of findings of Dupuytren's contracture of the palmar fascia has been suggested in AIDS patients without other predisposing factors (67). Fascial involvement results in flexion deformities at the metacarpophalangeal joints of the fingers. Its proposed pathogenesis via the destructive effects of oxidation by free radicals may be corroborated in this population, in whom free radicalization appears increased (68). Others have not found the prevalence of Dupuytren's in patients with HIV to vary significantly from that in the general population (69).

REFERENCES

1. Vandermolen LA, Fehir KM, Rice L. Multiple myeloma in a homosexual man with chronic lymphadenopathy. *Arch Int Med* 1985;145:745-746.
2. Karlsson A, Bratt G, Von Krogh G, Morfeldt-Manson L, Bottiger B, Sandstrom E. A prospective study of 115 initially asymptomatic HIV-infected gay men in Stockholm, Sweden. *Scand J Infect Dis* 1991;23(1):431-441.
3. Barbanera M, Menicagli V. Multiple myeloma in HIV infection. *Recenti Progressi in Medicina* 1990 Oct;81(10):663-665.
4. Monfardini S, Vaccher E, Pizzocaro G, Stellini R, Sinicco A, Sabbatani S, Marangolo M, Zagni R, Clerici M, Foa R. Unusual malignant tumors in 49 patients with HIV infection. *AIDS* 1989 Jul;3(7):449-452.
5. Karnad A, Wright J. Neoplastic complications of human immunodeficiency virus infection (Letter). *Am J Med* 1987;82:1282.

6. Karnad AB, Martin AW, Koh HK, Brauer MJ, Novich M, Wright J. Nonsecretory multiple myeloma in a 26-year-old man with acquired immunodeficiency syndrome, presenting with multiple extramedullary plasmacytomas and osteolytic bone disease. *Am J Hematol* 1989;32:305-310.
7. Voelkerding KV, Sandhaus LM, Kim HC, Wilson J, Chittenden T, Levine AJ, Raska K Jr. Plasma cell malignancy in the acquired immunodeficiency syndrome. Association with Epstein-Barr virus. *Am J Clin Pathol* 1989 Aug;92(2):222-228.
8. Shokunbi WA, Okpala IE, Shokunbi MT, Akinboye OD, Saliu I, Essien EM. Multiple myeloma coexisting with HIV-1 infection in a 65-year-old Nigerian man (Letter). *AIDS* 1991 Jan;5(1):115-116.
9. Israel AM, Kozinar B, Straus DJ. Plasmacytoma and the acquired immunodeficiency syndrome. *Ann Int Med* 1983;99:635-636.
10. von Keyserlingk H, Baur R, Stein H, Hoeffken G, Thiel E. Multiple myeloma in a patient at risk for AIDS. *Cancer Detect Prev* 1990;14(3):403-404.
11. Solomon L. Mechanisms of idiopathic osteonecrosis. *Orthop Clin N Am* 1985;16: 655-667.
12. Spencer JD, Brookes M. Avascular necrosis and the blood supply of the femoral head. *Clin Orthoped Relat Res* 1988 Oct;235:127-140.
13. Archer AG, Nelson MC, Abbondanzo SL, Bogumill GP. Case report 554. *Skeletal Radiol* 1989;18:380-384.
14. Gerster JC, Camus JP, Chave JP, Koeger AC, Rappoport G. Multiple site avascular necrosis in HIV infected patients. *J Rheumatol* 1991 Feb;18(2):300-302.
15. Goorney BP, Lacey H, Thurairajasingam S, Brown JD. Avascular necrosis of the hip in a man with HIV infection. *Genitour Med* 1990 Dec;66(6):451-452.
16. Martin-Crespo R, Escorihuela A, Soleto J, Gurbindo MD, Sampelayo T, Luque MR, Trevijano JL. Hip disease in AIDS children. *Intl Conf on AIDS* 1992 Jul 19-24;8(3):105.
17. Calabrese LH. Vasculitis and infection with the human immunodeficiency virus. In Winchester R (ed), AIDS and Rheumatic Disease. *Rheum Dis Clin North Am* 1991 Feb;17(1):1-195.
18. Beltran J. Infections and avascular necrosis. In Stark DD, Bradley WG (eds), *Magnetic Resonance Imaging*. St. Louis: C.V. Mosby, 1992.
19. D'Ambrosia RD, Shoji H, Riggins RS, Stadalnik RC, DeNardo GL. Scintigraphy in the diagnosis of osteonecrosis. *Clin Orthop Relat Res* 1978;130:139-143.
20. Glick M, Muzyka BC, Salkin LM. Acute hard and soft oral tissue destruction in HIV associated with low CD4+ counts. *Intl Conf on AIDS* 1992 Jul 19-24;8(2):B147.
21. Smith GL, Felix DH, Wray D. Current classifications of HIV-associated periodontal diseases. *Brit Dental J* 1993 Feb 6;174(3):102-105.
22. Tschakaloff A, Schahn E, Wagner W. Acute necrotizing bone destruction of the maxillary and mandibular midline area in HIV infection cases. *Deutsche Zeitschrift fur Mund-,Kiefer-, und Gesichts-Chirugie* 1989 Jul-Aug;13(1):249-251.

23. Levine RA, Glick M. Rapidly progressive periodontitis as an important clinical marker for HIV disease. *Compendium* 1991 Jul;12(7):478-482.
24. San Giacomo TR, Tan PM, Loggi DG, Itkin AB. Progressive osseous destruction as a complication of HIV-periodontitis. *Oral Surg Oral Med Oral Pathol* 1990 Oct;70(4): 476-479.
25. Quart AM, Small CB, Klein RS. Local destruction of labial surface of mandibular teeth by direct application of cocaine in drug users with AIDS. *Intl Conf on AIDS* 1989 Jun 4-9;5:471ts.
26. Wrzolek MA, Sher JH, Kozlowski PB, Rao C. Skeletal muscle pathology in AIDS: a pathology study. *Muscle and Nerve* 1990 Jun;13(6):508-515.
27. Wiley CA. Neuromuscular diseases of AIDS. *Faseb J* 1989 Nov 3;13:2503-2511.
28. Rosenblum M, Brew BJ, Aranow HJ, Hardy W, Cronin K, Price RW. Clinical-pathological features of HTLV-1 associated myelopathy (HAM) in AIDS. *Intl Conf on AIDS* 1989 Jun 4-9;5:457.
29. Dalakas M, Wichman A, Sever J. AIDS and the nervous system. *JAMA* 1989;261: 2396-2399.
30. Stern R, Gold J, DiCarlo EF. Myopathy complicating the acquired immune deficiency syndrome. *Muscle Nerve* 1987;10:318-322.
31. Lange DJ, Britton CB, Younger DS, Hays AP. The neuromuscular manifestations of human immunodeficiency virus infection. *Arch Neurol* 1988;45:1084-1088.
32. Neves O, Stein CM, Thornton C, Gangaidzo I, Thomas JE. Rhabdomyolysis associated with human immunodeficiency virus (HIV) infection. *Central African J Med* 1991 Nov;37(11):387-388.
33. Panegyres PK, Tan N, Kakulas BA, Armstrong JA, Hollingsworth P. Necrotising myopathy and zidovudine. (Letter), *Lancet* 1988;1:1050-1051.
34. Gorard DA, et al. Necrotizing myopathy and zidovudine. Letter, *Lancet* 1988; 1:1050.
35. Spence DW, Galantino ML, Mossberg KA, Zimmerman SO. Progressive resistance exercise: effect on muscle function and anthropometry of a select AIDS population. *Arch Phys Med Rehab* 1990 Aug;71(9):644-648.
36. Dalakas MC, Pezeshkpour GH, Gravell M, Sever JL. Polymyositis associated with AIDS retrovirus. *JAMA* 1986;256:2381-2383.
37. Nordstrom DM, Petropolis AA, Giorno R, et al. Inflammatory myopathy and acquired immunodeficiency syndrome. *Arth Rheumatol* 1989;32:475-479.
38. Chad DA, Smith TW, Blumenfeld A, et al. Human immunodeficiency virus (HIV)-associated myopathy: immunocytochemical identification of an HIV antigen (gp41) in muscle macrophages. *Ann Neurol* 1990 Oct;28(4):579-582.
39. Scelsi R, Lombardi M, Banfi P, Cosi V, Poggi P. Acquired rod-body myopathy associated with human immunodeficiency virus infection. *Ital J Neurolog Sci* 1990 Dec;11(6):609-613.
40. Dalakas MC, Pezeshkpour GH, Flaherty M. Progressive nemaline (rod) myopathy associated with HIV infection. (Letter), *NEJM* 1987;317:1602-1603.

41. Dalakas MC, Pezeshkpour GH. Neuromuscular diseases associated with human immunodeficiency virus infection. *Ann Neurol* 1981;23:538-548.
42. Gonzales MF, Olney RK, et al. Acute structural myopathy associated with human immunodeficiency virus infection. *Arch Neurol* 1988;45:585-587.
43. Marolda M, DeMercato R, Camporeale FS, Carandente M, Noce S, Cioffi M, Orsini AV, Cauli M, Bassi A. Myopathy associated with AIDS. *Ital J Neurol Sci* 1989 Aug;10(4):423-427.
44. Simpson DM, Wolfe DE. Neuromuscular complications of HIV infection and its treatment (Editorial). *AIDS* 1991 Aug;5(8):917-926.
45. Wallgren-Pettersson C, Kivisaari L, Jaaskelainen J, Lamminen A, Holmberg C. Ultrasonography, CT and MRI of muscles in congenital nemaline myopathy. *Pediatr Neurol* 1990 Jan- Feb;6(1):20-28.
46. Mitsui T, Miyata K, Kira J, Kobayashi T, Goto I. A case of adult-onset nemaline myopathy (adult-onset rod disease) with distal muscle hypertrophy. Risho Shinkeigaku. *Clin Neurol* 1991 May;31(5):546-549.
47. LaCroix C, Said G. Muscle siderosis in AIDS: a marker for macrophage dysfunction? *J Neurol* 1992 Jan;239(1):46-48.
48. Salzman L, Lee V, Grant P. Gallium uptake in myositis ossificans. *Clin Nucl Med* 1987;12(4):308-18.
49. DeSmet AA, Norris MA, Fisher DR. Magnetic resonance imaging of myositis ossificans: analysis of seven cases. *Skeletal Radiol* 1992;21(8):503-507.
50. Tamura S, Hasuo K, Kudo S, Uchino A, Yasumori K, Kawanami T, Masuda K. Atypical arteriographic features of myositis ossificans circumscripta (MOC). *Radiat Med* 1992 Jul-Aug;10(1):154-156.
51. Sud AM, Wilson MW, Mountz JM. Unusual clinical presentation and scintigraphic pattern in myositis ossificans. *Clin Nucl Med* 1992 Mar;17(3):198-199.
52. Nuovo MA, Norman A, Chumas J, Ackerman LV. Myositis ossificans with atypical clinical radiographic or pathologic findings: a review of 23 cases. *Skeletal Radiol* 1992;21(2):87-101.
53. Kransdorf MJ, Meis JM, Jelinek JS. Myositis ossificans: MR appearance with radiologic-pathologic correlation. *AJR* 1991 Dec;157(6):1243-1248.
54. Rooser B, Herrlin K, Rydholm A, Akerman M. Pseudomalignant myositis ossificans. Clinical, radiologic and cytologic diagnosis in 5 cases. *Acta Orthopaed Scand* 1989 Aug;60(4):457-460.
55. Amendola MA, Glazer GM, Agha FP, Francis IR, Weatherbee L, Martel W. Myositis ossificans circumscripta: CT diagnosis. *Radiology* 1983;149(3):775-779.
56. Drane WE, Tipler BM. Heterotopic ossification (myositis ossificans) in acquired immune deficiency syndrome. Detection by gallium scintigraphy. *Clin Nucl Med* 1987;12(5):433-435.
57. Shneerson JM. Digital clubbing and hypertrophic osteoarthropathy: the underlying mechanisms. *Brit J Dis Chest* 1981;75:113-129.

58. Hansen-Flaschen J, Nordberg J. Clubbing and osteoarthropathy. In Braman SS (guest ed), Pulmonary Signs and Symptoms. *Clin Chest Med* 1987;8:287-298.
59. Edeiken J, Dalinka M, Karasick D. *Roentgen Diagnosis of Diseases of Bone, 4th* ed. Baltimore: Williams and Wilkins, 1990.
60. Vaquer RA, Dunn EK, Bhat S, Heurich AE, Kamholz SL, Strashun AM. Reversible pulmonary uptake and hypertrophic pulmonary osteoarthropathic distribution of technetium-99m methylene diphosphonate in a case of *Pneumocystis carinii* pneumonia. *J Nucl Med* 1989 Sep;30(9):1563-1567.
61. Ali A, Tetalman MR, Fordham EW, Turner DA, Chiles JT, Patel SL, Schmidt KD. Distribution of hypertrophic osteoarthropathy. *AJR* 1980 Apr;134:771-780.
62. Pineda C. Diagnostic imaging in hypertrophic osteoarthropathy. *Clin Exper Rheum* 1992 May/Jun;10(Suppl 7):27-33.
63. Bhat S, Heurich AE, Vaquer RA, Dunn EK, Strashun AM, Kamholz SL. Hypertrophic osteoarthropathy associated with *Pneumocystis carinii* pneumonia in AIDS. *Chest* 1989 Nov;96(5):1208-1209.
64. Harris PJ. Hypertrophic pulmonary osteoarthropathy and human immunodeficiency virus (HIV). (Letter), *Ann Int Med* 1988 Aug 1;109(3):250.
65. Duro JC. Hypertrophic osteoarthropathy and the HIV (Letter). *Medicina Clinica* 1992 June;99(3):119.
66. Sabbagh M, Meyer O, DeBandt M, Salomen-Ceron D, Perronne C, Rosenblum W, Tremoliere F, Kahn MF. Bone manifestations associated with acquired immunodeficiency syndrome (AIDS). *Ann-Med-Interne(Paris)*1992;143(1):50-56.
67. Bower M, Nelson M, Gazzard BG. Dupuytren's contractures in patients infected with HIV. *Brit Med J* 1990 Jan;300(6718):164-165.
68. Baruchel S, Wainberg MA. The role of oxidative stress in disease progression in individuals infected by the human immunodeficiency virus. *J Leukocyte Biol 1992* Jul;52(1):111-114.
69. French PD, Kitchen VS, Harris JR. Prevalence of Dupuytren's contractures in patients infected with HIV. *Brit Med J* 1990 Oct 27;301(6758):967.

INDEX

Page numbers followed by the letter f refer to figures